Tails Along the Trails

Walking Adventures with Dogs

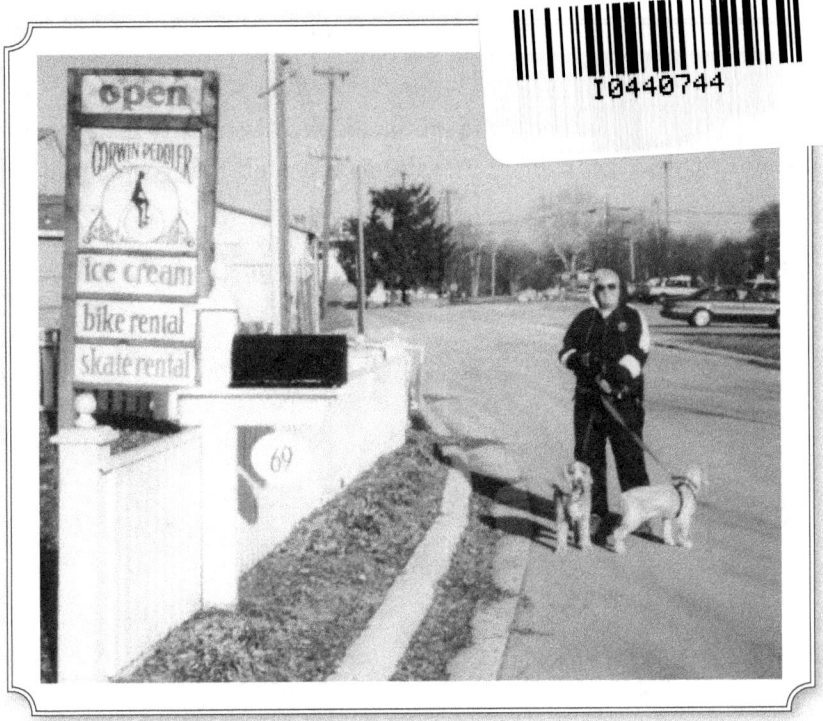

By Becky Corwin-Adams

Published by Brittdog Publishing

Tails Along the Trails by Becky Corwin-Adams

Published by Brittdog Publishing

Publishers Cataloging In Publication Data Available Upon Request

ISBN: 978-14839501-1-2

Contents

Dedication

This book is dedicated to my wonderful walking friends, Thelma and Judith. Many great memories were made while walking along the trails with the cocker spaniels and our friends.

Introduction

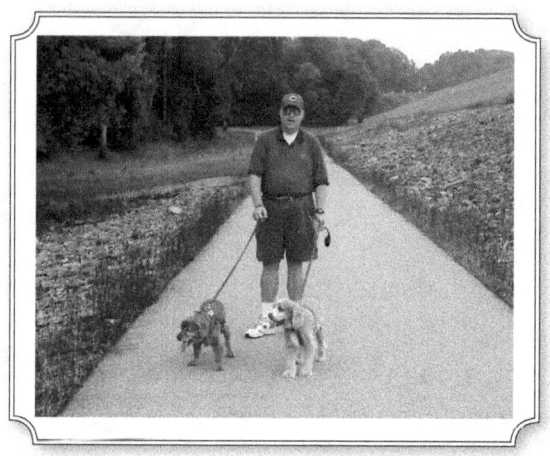

Barkley was a buff-and-white cocker spaniel who loved to walk. We rescued him from Defiance County (Ohio) Humane Society in 1998, when he was two years old. Barkley had very long legs and large paws. He was not a typical cocker spaniel. While most cocker spaniels have short, docked tails, Barkley had a long tail that went around in circles when he was happy.

My husband, Randy, and I are members of a walking club, the American Volkssport Association (www.ava.org). Volkssporting started in Germany. It is a personal fitness sports and recreation program offering noncompetitive walks, hikes, bike rides, swims, and cross-country skiing. Participants choose a time to start within the start/finish "window" and participate at their own pace.

We completed a 10-kilometer (six-mile) walk almost every weekend, and Barkley soon started joining us on our weekend walks. A few times, we walked 12 miles in one day, and Barkley didn't mind. When we went away for a weekend of walking, Barkley went along. He traveled all over Ohio, Indiana, Michigan, and Illinois to walk with us.

Barkley was our first volkssporting dog. We selected him to accompany us on our walks because he was the youngest and largest of our three cocker spaniels. Our vet once remarked that six miles was too far for a person to walk, let alone a dog! Barkley's first volkswalk was in Lima, Ohio, and we attended a walking club picnic and meeting after the walk. Barkley was six years old when he became a volkssporting dog.

Everyone who completes a walk gets an event stamp in their record book. Each of our cocker spaniels has their own Canine Event Book. Several of our cockers have at least six books filled with event stamps, totaling more than 200 walks.

Barkley had a walking buddy, a mixed-breed dog named Tootsie. Barkley got really excited when he saw Tootsie, and they walked very well together.

We soon started taking Brittany, our buff female cocker spaniel, on our walks in other cities and states. The first time we took Brittany along, our friend Thelma was very excited to meet her. We had previously explained to Thelma that Brittany did not like other female dogs, but Thelma opened the car door, took Brittany out, and tried to introduce her to Tootsie. We quickly had an altercation on our hands.

Barkley developed arthritis and gradually slowed down and started walking with a limp. The vet prescribed medication for the arthritis, but one day, Barkley could not finish a walk and had to be carried for the last three blocks. That was no easy feat, as Barkley weighed 41 pounds.

We took Bubba on some of our walks in his later years. After Bubba was successfully treated for heartworm disease at the age of two, our vet advised us not to take him on any walks longer than two miles. We took Bubba along on a few of our five-kilometer volkswalks and he did very well, so we started taking him more often, even when he was 13 years old.

Bubba loved roadkill: the deader, the better. On one of our walks, Thelma asked to walk Bubba. He soon picked up a very dead, flattened, crunchy squirrel from the side of the road. Thelma looked at me and asked what to do. I reminded her that the person holding the dog's leash was in charge, so she would have to deal with it. We continued to walk, with Bubba proudly carrying his treasure in his mouth, until he grew tired of it and dropped the nasty dead squirrel.

Celebrity Dogs on the Trail

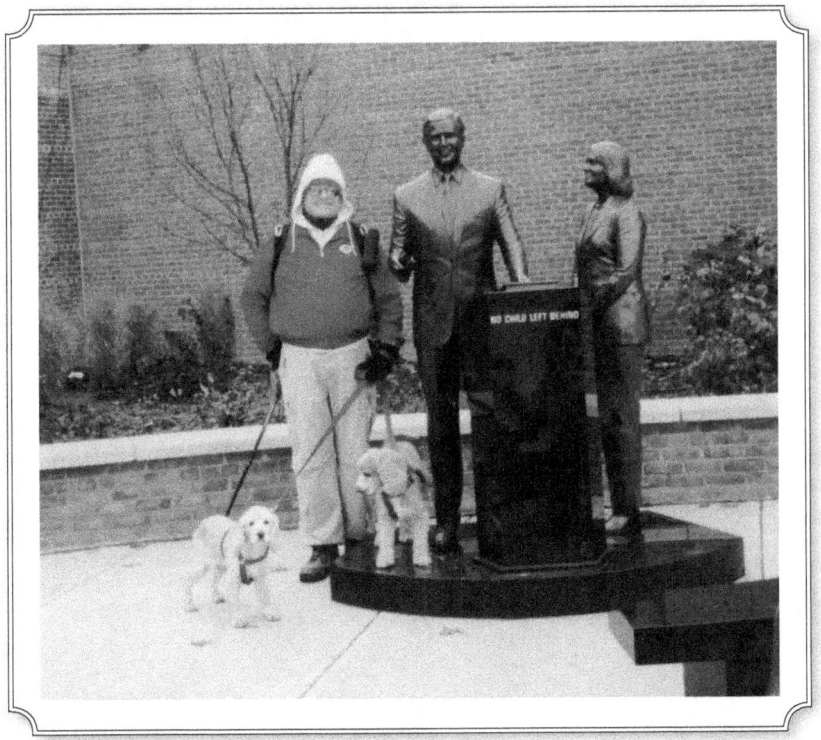

Barkley and Brittany accompanied us on a walk in Marion, Ohio, in the middle of their walking careers. A reporter from the Marion Star asked to interview the dogs after the walk. This is what she wrote:

> *There's history afoot in Marion. A walk and sight-see event visits the city and its monuments. However, people aren't the only ones who like a nice walk.*

Randy and Becky Adams took their dogs, Barkley and Brittany. It was Barkley's 101st 10-kilometer walk and Brittany's 59th. The Adams, of Bryan, are participants and organizers. Randy Adams is the president of the Ohio Volkssport Association and Becky Adams is the secretary.

Becky Adams said she doesn't just do it for the exercise. "We meet all of these wonderful people," she said, "We have walking friends we met from Dayton, Columbus, Cleveland. We know people from all over the state."

The article included photos of each of our dogs.

Charity Walks

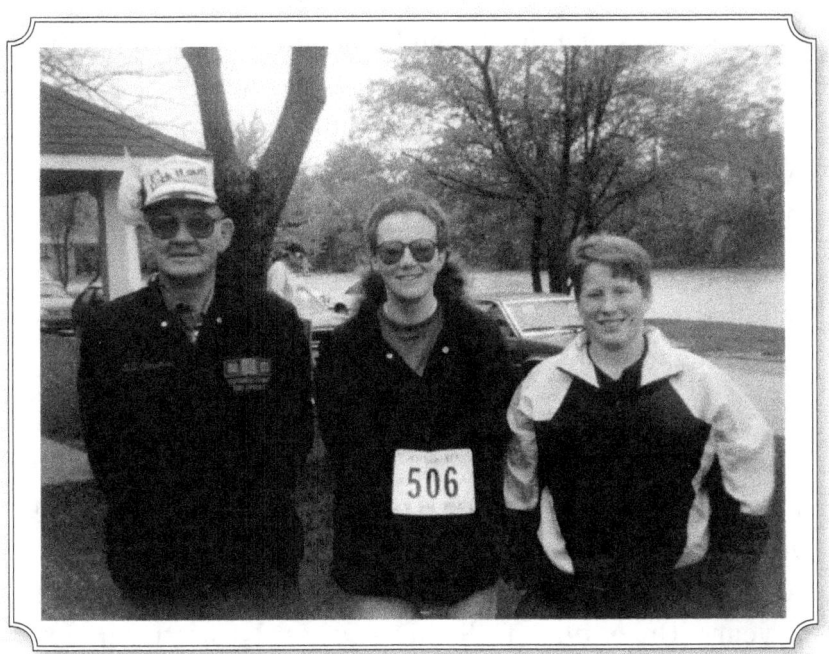

I participated in many charity walks in the '80s and '90s, in the early days of my walking career, before I learned about volkssporting.

I worked at Kmart for 17 years, and the company was the sponsor of March of Dimes Walk America. My first year as a member of the Walk America team was very memorable, since the event was 25 kilometers, the equivalent of 18 miles. We walked around Bryan, a small northwest Ohio town where Kmart 9000 and later, Kmart 3960 were located. Since it is such a small town, we walked many miles on gravel country roads. I was determined to finish the entire route, unlike many people who quit or cheated by skipping large parts of the trail.

I felt a great sense of accomplishment when I completed the walk. I was planning to go home and put my aching feet up, until one of my younger co-workers called in sick so that she could go to the lake. Being a glutton for punishment, I worked a six-hour shift at Kmart that evening, after walking 18 miles in less than six hours.

I participated in Walk America seven more times, including one year when I was accompanied by my young granddaughter and her mother.

In the late '80s, I joined the Bryan Parks and Recreation Department's walking club. Participants called the office monthly to log their walking miles, and at the end of each year, each club member received a tee shirt with their total miles on it. I earned dozens of these tee shirts over the next 25 years. Once, out of all those years, I was the number one walker for the year with 1,400 miles. My name and mileage often appeared in newspaper advertisements the following year.

The YWCA in Bryan opened in the late '80s and our family became members. The YWCA also had a walking club, and I walked hundreds of miles around the indoor track, where 12 laps equaled one mile. I worked at the front desk of the Y for a few years, and one of my responsibilities was keeping track of the walking club's mileage.

I also participated in St. Jude's three-mile walk in Defiance, my hometown, five times in the '90s. A family from my childhood church had a daughter, Kimberly, who was a patient at St. Jude's for several years, until she lost her valiant battle with childhood cancer. One year, my dad and my son walked with me, and it was a lot of fun to have three generations of walkers. Dad won a medal for first place in his age group that year.

Another benefit walk I participated in was a fundraiser for Angie, the young daughter of one of my co-workers at Kmart. Angie was born with serious health issues and later underwent a successful five-organ transplant. The five-mile pledge walk raised money to help with Angie's medical expenses. Angie passed away at the age of 26, and I will never forget her.

I once organized a fundraising walk for my church. Back in the early days of the computer age, the church was trying to raise money to purchase a computer system, and the walkathon money was added to the computer fund.

One of my favorite charities was the Community Pregnancy Center in Bryan. Each September, they held a six-mile walk to raise funds. I participated in this event 10 years in a row in the '90s. The walk mainly consisted of laps around the quarter-mile track at the Bryan Middle School. The live entertainment provided at the walk kept the 24 laps from becoming too boring.

Many small towns in northwest Ohio held festivals during the summer, and a walking event was often part of the festivities. I participated in many festival walks, including the three-mile Bryan Pepsi Run, the Montpelier Summer Fest five-kilometer walk, the Swamp Tromp five-kilometer walk at Sauder's Village in Archbold, the Defiance YMCA River Run two-mile walk, and the Sherwood Days five-kilometer walk.

I also participated in the West Unity Days five-kilometer walk, the Stryker Panther one-mile walk to raise money for a new school track, the Van Wert Hot Air Affair four-mile walk, and the Run for Lights at Ruihley Park in Archbold, a two-mile walk.

One of the most unusual walks I participated in was the Hicksville Hospital five-kilometer Fit Walk. The walk started at the hospital and ended downtown at a bandstand, where awards were given out. Participants were very upset to discover that the end of the walk was almost two miles away from the hospital parking lot. The walk ended up being a five-mile walk, on a very hot August day.

I participated in several more charity walks in the Bryan area: the Lutheran Social Services five-mile walk, the Bryan Fire Department Great Escapes three-mile walk, the Strides of Hope walk to benefit Cancer Assistance of Williams County, and the Williams County Making Strides Against Cancer five-mile walk. My son was a member of the Kmart team at the Strides of Hope walk, and he insisted on taking Brittany, our first cocker spaniel, along on the walk.

Three years in a row, I walked in the five-kilometer Walk, Roll or Run for Sarah's House, to raise funds for victims of domestic violence. I also participated in the Fountain City YWCA five-kilometer walk three times during my employment at the Y.

I was a member of my church team for the March 4 Jesus three-mile walk in Bryan two years in a row, the second time in pouring rain.

I joined two walking challenges while I was working at the YWCA: the 225-mile Exercise Across Ohio Challenge and the 2,777-mile Exercise Across America Challenge. I logged my miles and sent in my completed log sheets to receive a certificate of completion for these two events. I did some of the walking at the Y during inclement weather. Most of my walking was done outside, accompanied by Brittany and Bubba, our cocker spaniels.

I completed the Idita Walk, a virtual walk with minutes spent walking logged online, to coincide with the Iditarod Sled Dog Race in Nome, Alaska. Many of my walking friends also participated in the event.

After moving to Dayton in 2004, Randy and I walked in the Ghosts and Goblins five-mile Halloween walk around downtown Dayton. We decided that walking around Dayton in the dark of night is not the best thing to do, so we only participated one time.

The Ohio Road Runners Club sponsors an annual Turkey Trot on Thanksgiving morning in Miamisburg, Ohio. The five-mile race usually attracts over 6,000 runners and walkers. We have participated in the walk several times, including one year with our son, who is a runner. Randy's employer pays the registration fee for both of us, and we get a nice shirt every year. Some of the participants wear costumes, and it is always very entertaining. Since the route is an "out and back" trail, we pass most of the other participants at some point during the event.

Dog Attacks

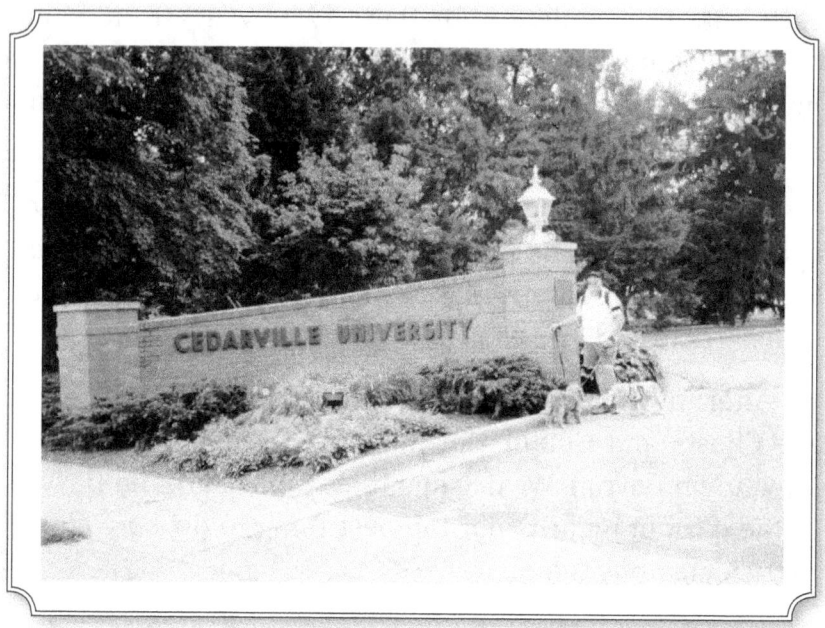

Dog attacks can be a serious problem for walkers. When we lived in Bryan, we had three encounters with dogs running loose, and each incident involved a Rottweiler.

Randy was attacked by a neighborhood Rottweiler while we were walking in our subdivision with our three cocker spaniels. The dog scaled a three-foot fence and approached us, barking and growling. He grabbed Barkley by the back of the neck and shook him like a rag doll. Mike, a neighbor, heard us yelling and ran down the street to assist. Mike bravely grabbed the Rottweiler by the collar and took him home, since he knew the owner.

Barkley ended up at the vet's office to be checked over, and he was fine. The owner received a citation and a small fine. She didn't learn anything from the incident, since the Rottweiler got loose about a year later and came charging at us again. This time, I was walking our three cocker spaniels by myself. The Rottweiler backed us up against a house and growled, forcing me to knock on the door of a stranger to ask for help. The police finally showed up, and the cockers and I were able to walk home. We weren't harmed, just badly frightened. Once again, the owner was fined for dog-at-large.

The third, and most serious incident, occurred less than a year later. It was a warm spring day, and we decided to take the three cocker spaniels on a long walk along a bike path in our neighborhood. A man had left a large Rottweiler on a tie out that was secured in the ground with a small tent stake, before going out of town for the day. The dog easily pulled the tent stake out of the rain-soaked ground, crossed a busy highway, and started growling at our cockers.

I started to walk away with our dogs, as Randy tried to control the Rottweiler. He was bitten 21 times on the right hand and both arms, as traffic passed by on the highway, without anyone stopping to help. The Rottweiler finally got tired and went home. We walked more than a mile back to our house: me with the three cocker spaniels, Randy dripping blood and very pale, close to going into shock.

We went to the emergency room, and the county dog warden was called. She refused to go into the treatment room to talk to Randy or to look at his wounds. The dog warden refused to cite the owner, even though it is a felony the first time a dog attacks a human or another animal. The law is there, but the enforcement isn't!

We phoned the owner to discuss the medical bills, and he told us to contact his lawyer, right before he slammed down the phone. We eventually contacted a lawyer and filed a lawsuit, since the dog owner had no interest in resolving the case. We later learned that the dog owner was a county employee and a friend of the dog warden, a case of the "good old boy" syndrome. We finally settled the case out of court, after it went on for nearly two years. We also learned, from a family member employed at a vet's office, that the Rottweiler had been euthanized 10 days after the attack.

Next Generation of Dogs

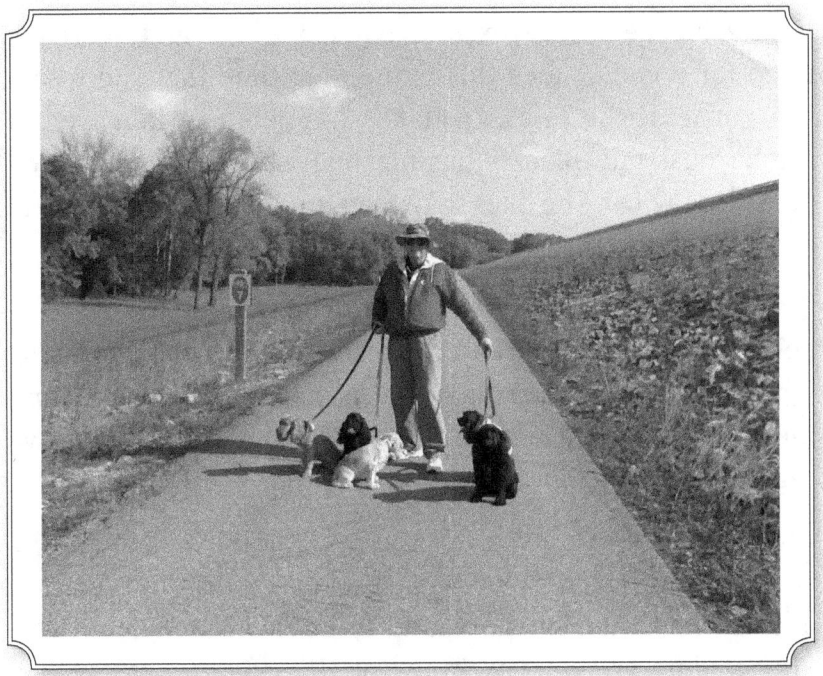

Brittany and Barkley completed hundreds of volkswalks with us. After they passed away, we adopted some younger cocker spaniels and soon started taking them along on our walks.

We adopted Blackie as a puppy. She is a good long distance walker, so she accompanies us on most of our volkswalks. Blackie completed her first volkswalk in Bradford, Ohio. Her volkssporting career began the first week she lived with us.

On one of Blackie's first walks, she encountered a large bronze statue of a lion along the trail. Blackie was afraid of the statue and growled at it. She must have thought it was a big dog.

Blackie gets very excited when we are getting ready to go for a walk. Since this is the only time that she wears her harness, she knows what is happening when we get the harness out. Blackie has her own special, bone-shaped pillow in the car. She likes to nap on the way to a walk so that she will have plenty of energy to walk 10 kilometers.

Blackie gets so excited when we arrive at the starting point that she makes "happy noises." Everyone at the start table knows she is coming because they hear Blackie before they see her. Blackie waits, very impatiently, while we register for the event.

Blackie calms down after the first kilometer or so of the walk. She walks at a steady pace. If it is warm out, Blackie likes to lie down in the shade to cool off along the trail. Checkpoints are very exciting, too. Blackie knows she will be getting a drink and possibly a treat. Blackie does not like community water bowls, so she can sometimes be seen drinking water out of a paper cup at a checkpoint.

Blackie loves to walk with her Aunt Thelma. Blackie's most important job is pulling Thelma up the hills. Sometimes, Blackie gets confused and tries to pull Thelma down the hills at a fast pace. When we stop to use the restroom along the trail, Blackie whines the entire time and stares at the restroom door until we come out. Blackie walks with us so much that a lot of people know her by name.

Sometimes we stop for a picnic lunch after a walk. Blackie usually takes a nap under the picnic table. She also likes to sleep in the car on the way home from a walk.

Blackie has completed walks in Ohio and Indiana. Some of her favorite walks are those associated with festivals. Blackie loves popcorn, and many of the festival walks have popcorn for sale. Blackie knows we will buy some popcorn to share with her after the walk.

One cool autumn day, we left Blondie and Blackie in the car after we took them on a long walk. While we had lunch with Thelma, Blondie destroyed the door panel of the car. She even chewed on the shoulder harness.

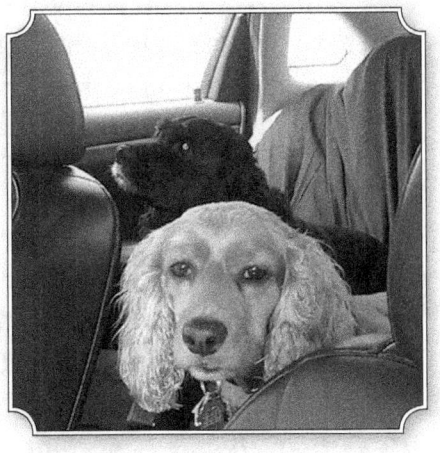

Another time, we left Blackie and Blondie in the car while we went inside to order a pizza after a walk. When we returned five minutes later, they had eaten half a bag of buttered popcorn. The bag was on the floor of the car. Both girls were fastened in with harnesses and seat belts, but Blondie had managed to reach the bag, open it, and share it with Blackie. Blondie's stomach looked like much larger than usual, so she couldn't deny her evil deed.

Blondie and Betsy walked with us for several years. Betsy's first volkswalk was at Riverbend Park in Findlay, Ohio, and she was very excited to meet a lot of new people. Betsy jumped up on the table where brochures for upcoming walks were displayed, and the brochures went flying everywhere. Betsy jumped on the table several more times before the day was over.

On one of her first volkswalks, Betsy suddenly vomited and fell down on the sidewalk. After lying there for a few minutes, she jumped up and started walking again. We didn't think too much about the incident, until Betsy began having infrequent seizures a few years later. That episode was more than likely a seizure, although we didn't realize it at the time, since it was not like the seizures Brittany and Bubba had for many years.

On one of our walks, Blondie noticed a two-foot-tall metal rooster in a yard and really wanted to attack it. It was too close to the house to let her inspect it, but she really enjoyed barking and growling at it.

On another walk, Blondie saw a large cat sitting in the middle of the sidewalk. The cat refused to move, so we tried to walk past it. The cat lunged at Blondie, the smallest of the three cocker spaniels accompanying us that day. Randy had to hit the mean cat with his walking stick, and it finally left Blondie alone. We stopped to see if Blondie was okay, and we noticed one of the cat's claws was stuck in Blondie's cheek, so we removed it and continued our walk.

Blondie never liked cats after that incident, so we often crossed the street to avoid them. Blondie wanted to attack every cat she saw. More than seven years after the cat incident, Blondie became friends with Highway, the resident cat at our vet's office.

Blondie and Betsy are smaller cockers with short legs, and they really did not enjoy walking six miles. Blondie had been a puppy mill mom for three years and had never been outside until she came to live with us. Her paws would bleed on some of our longer walks, since they were so sensitive.

After we adopted Brandon and Beezus, two younger cockers with longer legs, they started accompanying us, along with Blackie, on most of our walks.

Brandon's first volkswalk was at Huffman MetroPark in Dayton. Near the end of the walk, Brandon lay down in the middle of the trail and refused to get up. After a brief rest period, he was ready to finish the walk. Brandon was only one year old at the time.

Brandon has a special friend, Helga, who always wants to take him home with her. I'm not sure if it is Brandon she is enamored with, or the purple collar he wears, since Helga's favorite color is purple. On several occasions, I offered to find a dog like Brandon for Helga to adopt, since I am very involved with cocker rescue. I think Helga would prefer to "dognap" Brandon.

Beezus' first volkswalk was at Jungle Jim's Market in Fairfield, Ohio. We had arranged to meet Barb, a friend from my online cocker spaniel forum, at the market. Barb lived nearby, and we also met her husband Bill and their cockers, Gracie and Ginger. Beezus was very wild and crazy that day, and she was anxious to start her first volkswalk.

Volkssporting

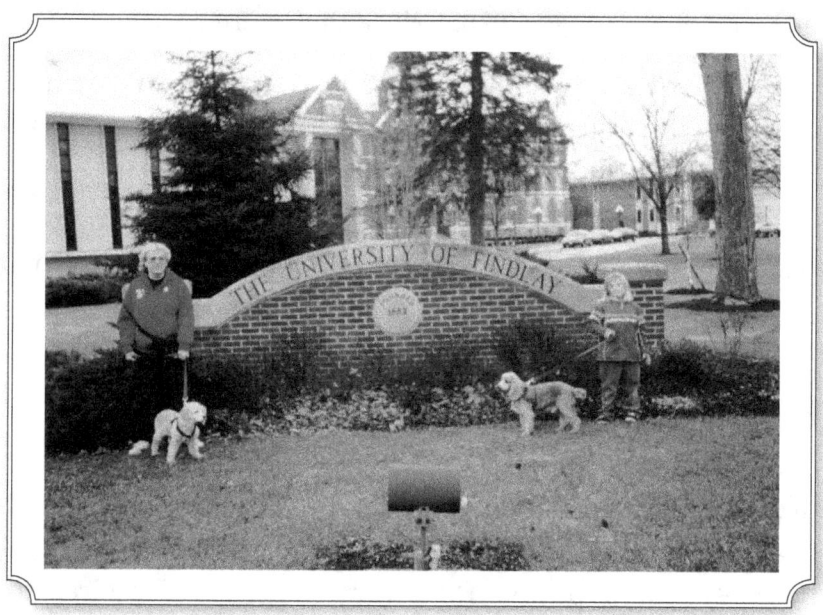

Walking, also called "volksmarching," is the most popular of all the volkssporting activities. Volkssporting in the United States is sponsored by the American Volkssport Association (AVA), which has a nationwide network of about 300 active clubs offering more than 3,000 volkssporting events each year.

The AVA was founded in 1976. It is a nonprofit 501(c)3 corporation dedicated to promoting fun, fitness, and friendship. Volkssporting events take place throughout the country, all year round. Historic and scenic sites are selected, and trails are carefully laid out and marked, with directions or maps provided. The designated start point is open for several hours to allow participants to begin their volkssporting adventure at their leisure. Trails along the route have checkpoints, which are monitored for safety and security. Participants often gather at the finish point to talk with friends and enjoy some light refreshments.

Year-round walks are also available. Unlike traditional volkssport events, which are limited to one day with a set start and finish time, a year-round event is open daily, January through December. At the event start, a participant must register in the log book, sign the waiver, and obtain a start card. Directions and maps are provided, and participants can complete the trail at their leisure.

Most participants purchase record books to keep track of their accomplishments. There are books to record the number of events completed and the number of kilometers walked. Completed books can be sent to the AVA headquarters to receive awards, including certificates, patches, and hat pins.

My First Volkswalk

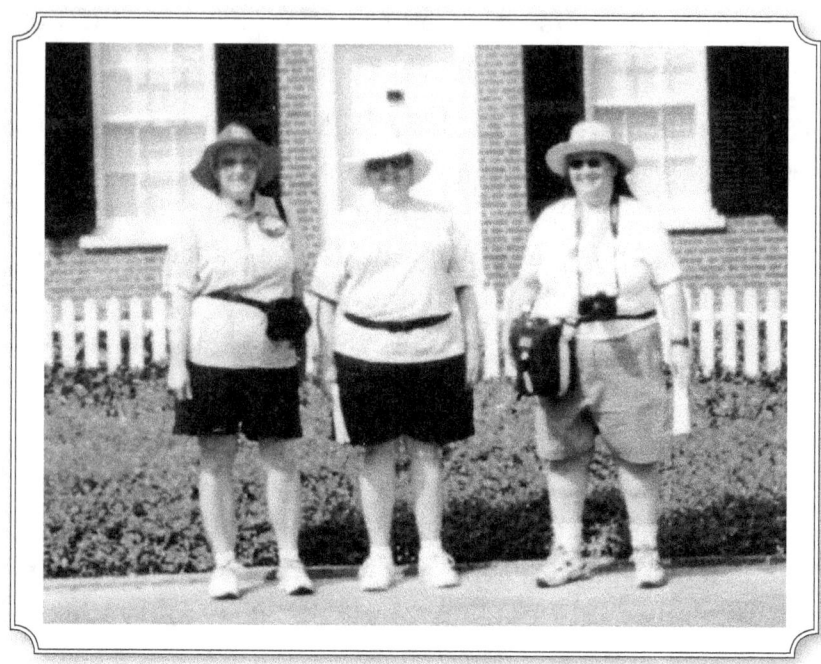

My first volkswalk was in September 1997. Randy was out of town for the weekend, and I was bored. I heard about a "free" walk at Harrison Lake State Park and decided to check it out. The people at the start table were very helpful, and I noticed that the people along the trail were very friendly, too.

I started out planning to walk the five-kilometer route. After completing the shorter route, I was feeling so good that I decided to complete the other half of the 10-kilometer trail. The first five-kilometer trail went around the lake in one direction. The second trail involved walking in the opposite direction around the lake.

After the walk, Kitty and Virginia, the ladies at the finish table, explained volkssporting to me and gave me some brochures. I decided to buy a new walker packet, since it was only five dollars. There was another walk the following day in Bryan, where we lived at the time.

The walk in Bryan was my second volkswalk. I walked with a very nice couple and their five-year-old son. They had participated in volkssporting in Germany and were just getting back into walking in the States. I learned a lot about the sport from this friendly couple.

The following weekend, Randy experienced his first volkswalk. I had wanted to explore volkssporting further, so I found a walk nearby, in Auburn, Indiana. We drove to the Auburn-Cord-Duesenberg Museum where the walk started. We bought record books for Randy at that time, although he didn't think he could complete a 10-kilometer walk, and I wasn't sure he could, either.

I discovered that the walk was actually 11 kilometers, but I didn't tell Randy, since I thought that extra kilometer would be enough to make him change his mind about participating. We did complete the walk, and the rest is history. Randy still mentions the fact that I tricked him into walking 11 kilometers on his first volkswalk. We have each completed more than 900 volkssport events, in 27 states and Canada.

Trail Trolls

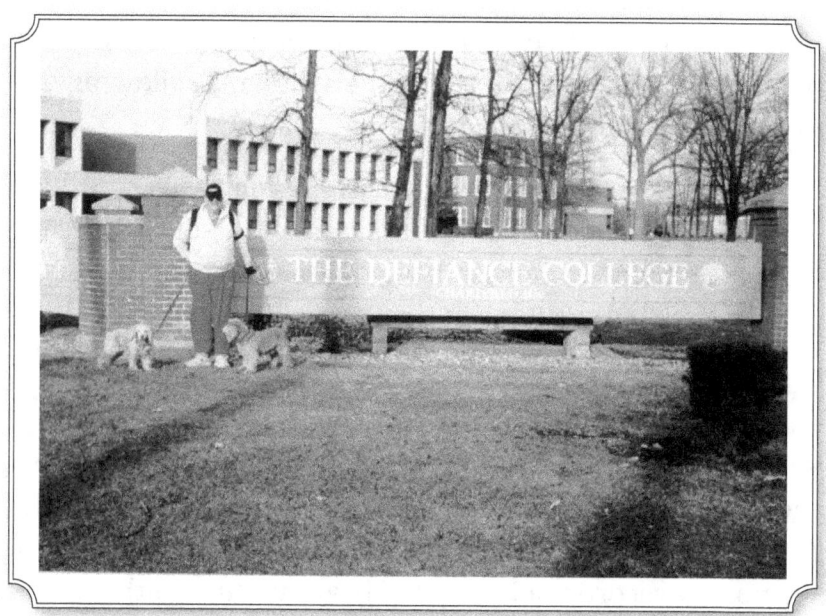

We started our own walking club, Trail Trolls, a volkssport associate club. At the time, we lived in Bryan, and there were no clubs closer than an hour away. I had a collection of more than 500 Troll dolls, dating back to the '60s, so we decided to include "trolls" in our club name. We set up some walking trails in the area, and we walked those trails many times each year.

Our Bryan volkswalk started at Lester's Diner (now Four Seasons Diner), on the main street of the "Fountain City." Lester's was a '60s-style diner, modeled after Mel's Diner on the television program, "Alice." The trail continued through several of Bryan's beautiful city parks, including Garver Park, Moore Park, Recreation Park, and Mattie Marsh Park.

The trail also went through Bryan's beautiful, quaint downtown area and past the Williams County Courthouse. During the Christmas season, the downtown area is a holiday wonderland with splendid light displays around the courthouse square. Thousands of Christmas lights, a large nativity set, a huge snowman, and Santa's Workshop are all located on the square. Volunteers decorate the square six weeks before Christmas, creating one of the largest and best Christmas light displays in the state of Ohio.

Another of our club's trails was in Defiance, my birthplace and hometown. The trail went past the Defiance County Courthouse, the campus of Defiance College, and through a historic cemetery with burial sites of War of 1812 veterans. The highlight of the Defiance walk was the grounds of Fort Defiance, built by General "Mad" Anthony Wayne, on the banks of the Maumee River. The Defiance Public Library, a historic Carnegie library, was later built at the site of Fort Defiance.

The historic trail also goes through Pontiac Park, the birthplace of Ottawa Indian Chief Pontiac, born in 1712. We also walked past Miami and Erie Canal Lock 5. My favorite part of the walk was the historic home district on Holgate Avenue.

Trail Trolls also created a trail in Archbold, starting at historic Sauder's Village. Dozens of structures, built by hand a century earlier, were moved from locations throughout northwest Ohio to create the village. The buildings and craft studios are staffed by craftsmen working in traditional arts, displaying their skills for visitors.

The trail continued into downtown Archbold, along the beautiful, tree-shaded streets of the small town. A highlight of the trail was Ruihley Park, which also had a wonderful holiday light display.

Our club also created a trail in Montpelier, a small village in Williams County. The trail started at the Williams County Fairgrounds, passed by the historic 1860 George Lett log house and an old Wabash railroad caboose, and ran across a wooden bridge replica. We crossed an elevated bridge over railroad tracks in the middle of our walk and found an ice cream shop and a beautiful city park at the foot of the bridge. There are many historic homes and business in downtown Montpelier.

Our club later took over several walks from another club that disbanded. One of the walks was in Lima, with two different trails. One trail went along the river walk, which was often flooded, and the other trail was in downtown Lima. There is a nut shop downtown, and Randy liked to stop there and buy some nuts to eat as he walked.

On one of our walks, Randy started having chest pains after eating the nuts. The trail started at a hospital, so halfway through the walk, Randy ended up in the emergency room. After monitoring him for several hours, doctors determined that he just had a bad case of indigestion. As soon as he was released, Randy wanted to finish the walk, but I informed him that we were done walking that day.

Another of our club's walks was in New Bremen, along the Miami and Erie Canal. We also created a walk in nearby St. Marys, a small town along the Auglaize River. Randy's grandparents lived in St. Marys for a few years, so we were very familiar with the town. There was an interesting flea market downtown in the former G.C. Murphy's building, and we usually stopped there after our walk.

One of Barkley's first walks was in St. Marys, and we forgot to bring a water bowl for him. We stopped at a thrift shop along the walk route and bought a green plastic bowl for 25 cents. We used that bowl for many years, and I still have it. I could never throw it away, and we always refer to it as "Barkley's bowl."

Our club also had a walk in Wapakoneta; this trail passed by the Armstrong Air and Space Museum and the boyhood home of Neil Armstrong. My friend Judith knew a man in Wapakoneta with a very interesting home, and we had the opportunity to tour the back yard on one of our walks. The man had collected lots of old bowling balls in various colors and used them for landscaping. The back yard contained walls made of rock, lots of foliage, and an old stone building.

Outings Across Ohio

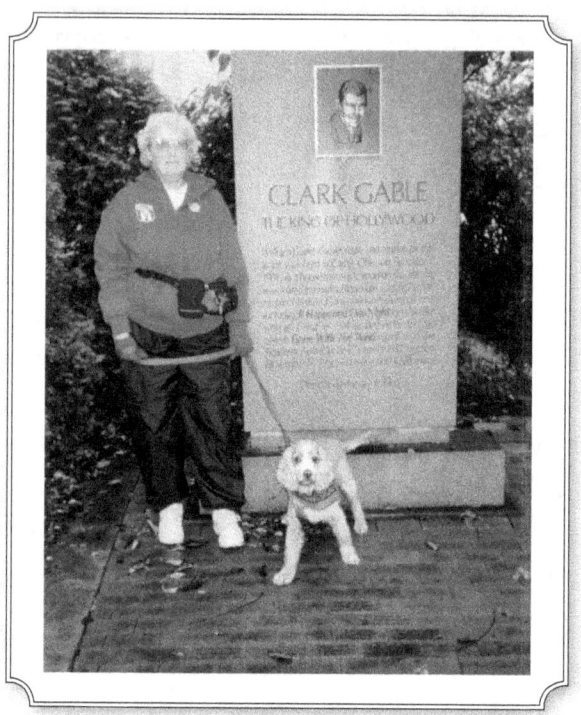

We completed many walks in different parts of Ohio while trying to reach our goal of walking in each of Ohio's 88 counties. One of the most interesting walks took place in Marietta. Barkley accompanied us on this very historic walk. We saw many unique wood carvings, beautiful murals, and the riverboat, Becky Thatcher, along the trail.

Another interesting walk was held in Dresden, home of the Longaberger basket factory. Barkley also went on this walk, and we stopped for a photo in front of the world's largest Longaberger basket at the company's headquarters.

In Bexley, a suburb of Columbus, we walked past the governor's mansion and around the campus of Capital University. We had never visited the state capital, even though we were lifelong residents of Ohio.

Another Columbus walk took us around the campus of Ohio State University. It was a birthday walk planned by Bob, a walker who had recently retired from the University. In one of the buildings, we stopped for birthday cake and a large selection of snack foods.

We had two interesting dog encounters at walking events in two parks in Columbus. The first was on a cold January day. At the beginning of the walk, Brittany and Barkley were very interested in a small, white dog that was running loose. The dog suddenly jumped into a small pool with a fountain. Then the dog's owner jumped in, fully clothed, to save the dog.

The second incident happened in the parking lot of another Columbus park. We were walking with Brittany, Barkley, and our friend Thelma. We noticed a man ahead of us walking two large dogs. He took them to his car, opened the trunk, put the dogs inside, closed the trunk, and drove off. We stared at the car for a few seconds, stunned, not sure if we should call the police. We opted not to, since we didn't know the phone number and really didn't want to dial 911.

Another interesting walk was in Cadiz, where we saw a lot of murals and passed by Clark Gable's home. We also saw some interesting murals in Washington Court House.

In southeast Ohio, we completed walks in Waynesville and Corwin, two small, historic towns that are in close proximity to one another. I was especially interested in visiting Corwin, a village named for some of my ancestors. The walk started at The Corwin Peddler ice cream shop and took us along a busy bike trail. Brittany, Bubba, and Barkley accompanied us on these walks several times.

One snowy winter day, we walked in Waynesville with Barkley and Blackie. I slipped on the icy wooden bridge when the cocker spaniels decided they needed to go faster than I was walking. I knew that the bridge was slippery, since I had already walked over it once, so I anticipated the problem and was able to control the fall, so I was not injured.

We walked at John Bryan State Park in Yellow Springs on a sunny spring day. It was the year the 17-year locusts appeared in Ohio. Brittany and Barkley did not pay much attention to the locusts. There were thousands of locusts along the trail, and they crunched when we stepped on them. We had never seen anything like it.

Fortunately, we left Bubba at home that day. He would have enjoyed eating as many live locusts as he could. Bubba loved bugs and would catch cicadas and locusts in our back yard. He did not even bother to kill them. He just swallowed them alive, in one gulp. You could still hear them buzzing inside of him.

The city of Versailles had a poultry festival every summer. We enjoyed that walk very much and stopped for a picnic lunch of barbecued chicken halfway through the walk. One time we took Barkley and Brittany along, and we found a picnic table in a secluded area so the dogs could relax. Soon, a family with some annoying children sat at the next table. Those unruly kids could not leave our tired dogs alone, even after we asked politely, so we ended up cutting our picnic short.

One very cold day, we walked in Bluffton with our friend Judith. We were all wearing many layers of clothing to stay warm. Randy got too close to the edge of the trail and fell. He didn't try to stop himself as he rolled down to the bottom of the hill. Judith and I watched his descent down the hill and were amazed when he stood up, laughing and uninjured.

A few years later, we walked at a park in Bluffton with Brittany and Barkley. After the walk was a club meeting that lasted for several hours. The tired dogs slept through the entire meeting. Sadly, Brittany passed away in her sleep six days later. Every time we drive past that park, Randy reminds me that Brittany went on her last volkswalk there.

In the Toledo area, we often walked in Maumee and Perrysburg. In the heart of downtown Perrysburg, we walked past a statue of Commodore Oliver Hazard Perry, after whom Perrysburg is named. There was a wonderful ice cream shop at the end of the Maumee trail, and we always stopped for ice cream after the walk.

We walked in nearby Grand Rapids, and the trail went along the canal and past Ludwig Mill and a historic log cabin. Canal boats, drawn by mules, offered rides every hour during the summer.

In Milan, we walked past Thomas Edison's birthplace. In Eaton, we met a man along the trail who told us the history of the covered bridge he had helped to restore. Fort Saint Clair, also on the Eaton trail, has a historic cemetery. In December, there is a wonderful holiday light display at the fort.

We walked in Oxford, around the campus of Miami University several times with Barkley, Blackie, and Blondie. It was an enjoyable walk for the dogs, since many of the college students stopped to pet them. Blondie especially thrived on the attention. We were sitting on a brick wall on campus, taking a break, when Blondie suddenly jumped off the back of the wall. The drop was several feet, and we had trouble getting her back up the embankment.

Brittany, our first cocker, had done the same thing years earlier during a walk in Defiance. Blondie was a miniature of our first cocker, and we always thought Brittany was telling her to behave in certain ways. We were sure Brittany told Blondie to jump over that wall!

Bubba, along with Blackie and Blondie, completed 10-kilometer volkswalks in Maria Stein, Lewisburg, and Carriage Hill MetroPark in Huber Heights. Bubba did very well for a 13-year-old cocker who had not started long distance walking until he was older.

Bubba, Blackie, Blondie, and Betsy all accompanied us on a walk in Mechanicsburg. We saw a big, dead frog, with a long, red tongue hanging out. I was lucky to steer Bubba away from it, since he was the extremely fond of roadkill.

A very challenging walk was at Charleston Falls near Tipp City. Randy had to carry Blackie and Blondie over stepping stones across a creek, three times. When we came to a very large hill, I suggested we go back the other way, but Randy insisted that we go up that hill. I had already taken a tumble on level ground at the beginning of the walk. The combination of the two dogs pulling me, the wet grass, and a small hole I stepped in caused me to gracefully fall down on my knees. Several people noticed the mud and asked what happened. After my fall, Randy would not allow me to carry the dogs over the creek.

Wild Weather Walks

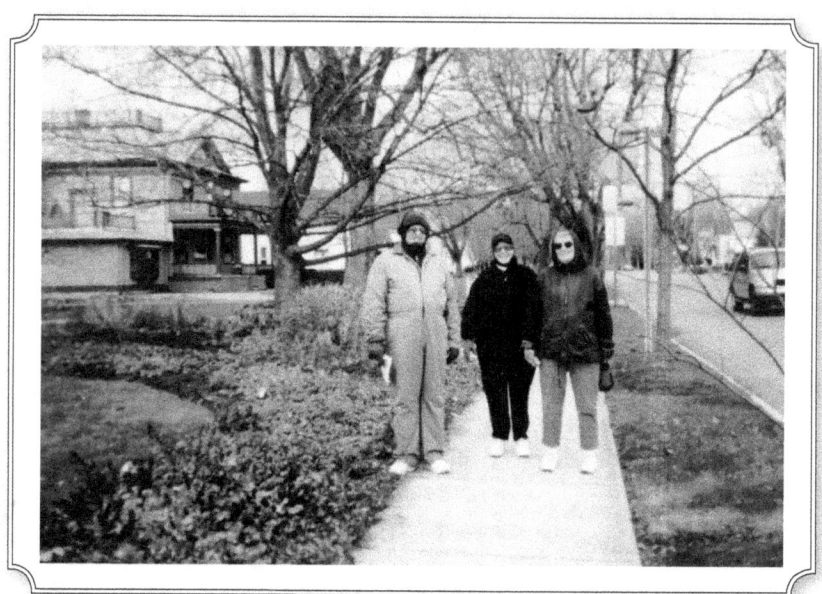

We completed some of our walks in very nasty weather. As dedicated walkers who often traveled long distances to walk, we didn't let bad weather stop us from completing a walk.

One of our most memorable Ohio walks was at the Voice of America Park in West Chester. This 435-acre park was originally a part of the Voice of America-Bethany Relay Station. The park features a 35-acre lake encircled by a 1.4-mile paved multi-purpose path. We walked around that lake five times, on a very cold, windy, rainy day. By the end of our walk, the rain had turned to snow.

Our new walking friend Cindy retreated to the car to wait for us after the first loop around the lake. Thelma borrowed Randy's golf umbrella, and the wind quickly turned it inside out and destroyed it. We took Barkley and Brittany to the car to warm up after several loops around the lake. We had driven three hours for the sole purpose of completing a 10-kilometer walk, and we were determined to finish. Just like the United States Postal Service, we would not be stopped by rain, sleet, or snow. This walk offered all three!

Another very miserable walk was in South Charleston, Ohio, during a hard, steady rain. After the first half of the walk, we were soaking wet clear up to our waists, so we decided not to finish the last five kilometers of the walk.

One rainy spring day, our friend Judith joined us for a walk at Kensington Park in Milford, Michigan. Halfway through the walk, a bad storm arrived suddenly, with intense thunder and lightning. Already soaking wet, we took shelter in the next picnic pavilion we came to. It was very scary situation, until the storm finally passed, and we were able to continue our walk, in spite of being very cold and wet. Fortunately, the dogs had stayed home that day.

We were members of a walking club in Fort Wayne, Indiana, for a few years. One very rainy evening, we were putting up trail markers for a walk the following day. The man in charge of marking the trail seemed to be confused about where the trail actually was. Every time we questioned him, he replied, "Trust me." We always referred to him as "Mr. Trust Me" after that experience.

The trail soon became muddy and slippery, and we encountered a lady who had fallen in the park. After finding a police officer to assist her, we continued on our mission. We later realized that the police officer had been following us through the park, removing the markers we were putting up. We had to go back and re-mark a portion of the trail.

We had a similar trail marking experience in Richmond, Indiana, a few years later. We offered to help Thelma mark a trail on a rainy evening. At one point, the rain became very heavy, and we were forced to take shelter in a picnic pavilion. The trail went sharply downhill near the pavilion and the rain quickly flooded the trail. We had to wait almost an hour until the rain stopped and the water receded, before we could continue walking. Fortunately, we never took any of the cocker spaniels along when we were marking a trail.

Holiday Walks

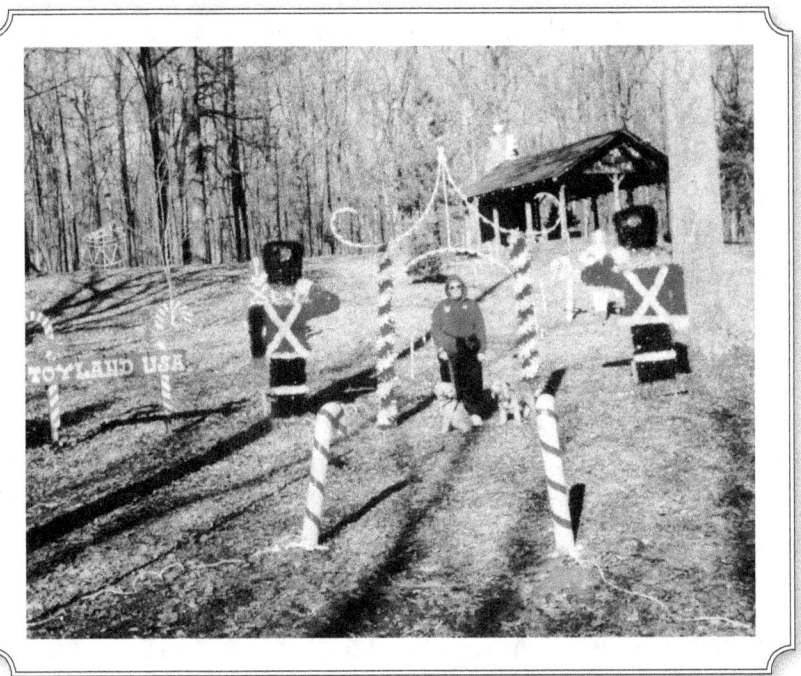

Every year, there is a holiday walk in Springboro in conjunction with a Christmas festival. Most of our cocker spaniels have completed this walk at least once. We took four dogs along one time—Bubba, Blackie, Blondie, and Betsy. We had planned to leave Bubba at home, but he really wanted to go along, and he did very well for a 13-year-old dog.

Betsy and Blondie conspired to trip Randy in the middle of the walk. He very gracefully rolled over a curb and didn't fall on any of the dogs. I had seen the fall coming, but there was nothing I could do to prevent it. Betsy thought it was a game, so she jumped on him and licked his face as he lay on the ground.

Near the end of the trail was the festival, which was interesting to walk through with four dogs. The cocker spaniels were on their best behavior, for once, and they really enjoyed the kettle corn booth. The cockers cleaned up all of the popcorn on the ground, and we bought a big bag of kettle corn to eat later. We arrived at the festival in the middle of the parade, so it was a very challenging walk. There were two Clydesdales and two miniature ponies in the parade. The cockers ignored them, unlike Brittany, our first cocker spaniel, who would have barked and growled at the horses.

A few years earlier, we had taken Barkley and Brittany on two Christmas walks. Both walks had live nativity scenes along the trail. At each walk, Brittany got close to a cow and growled in its face. We got nasty looks from some of the people, as we quickly pulled our fearless cocker spaniel away.

One year, during a series of Christmas walks in downtown Cincinnati, Randy stopped to use the restroom in a downtown restaurant. He pushed on the door repeatedly while someone inside was trying to hold the door closed. Finally, Randy managed to open the door and discovered a homeless man and woman inside of the restroom. The man told Randy to leave because the couple was "trying to have a private moment." Randy waited patiently outside until the couple finished their "private moment" and exited the restroom.

After one of the walks, we had dinner at a winery, a private party just for the walkers. The invitations stated, "adults only," but one couple brought along their unruly four-year-old daughter, who ran around the dining room, bothering everyone.

We also completed a Christmas walk in downtown Indianapolis several times. We took Barkley and Brittany along, and the only way to get to the starting point of the walk, in the lobby of a large hotel, was to take the elevator from the parking garage. We soon learned that Brittany was terrified of elevators, and we got some nasty looks from other passengers who didn't think dogs should be allowed on the elevator.

On New Year's Eve of the New Millennium (2000) we completed two walks in Middletown. The first walk started before midnight, and the second walk started after midnight. We planned to do the shorter walk, the five-kilometer trail, of each event since it was cold, snowy, and so late at night. The first walk seemed to be taking longer than planned, as we followed the written directions we had been given. We finally realized we were almost done with the 10-kilometer walk. The directions included a line at the very bottom of the page that gave special instructions about where to turn around for the shorter trail.

It was a three-hour drive home to Bryan, and we slept most of New Year's Day, instead of doing the walk in Columbus as we had planned. Most people were hung over from drinking, but we were hung over from walking!

One unseasonably warm New Year's Day, we went to Westerville, a suburb of Columbus, to walk-in the New Year with our friends Thelma, Ginny, and Jackie. Brittany and Barkley accompanied us, along with Barkley's canine walking buddy, Tootsie. Part of the trail went through a park with a very muddy soccer field. We tried to avoid the worst of the mud, but Brittany managed to get covered with it, so we had to give her a bath when we got home.

The Cockers' Favorite Walks

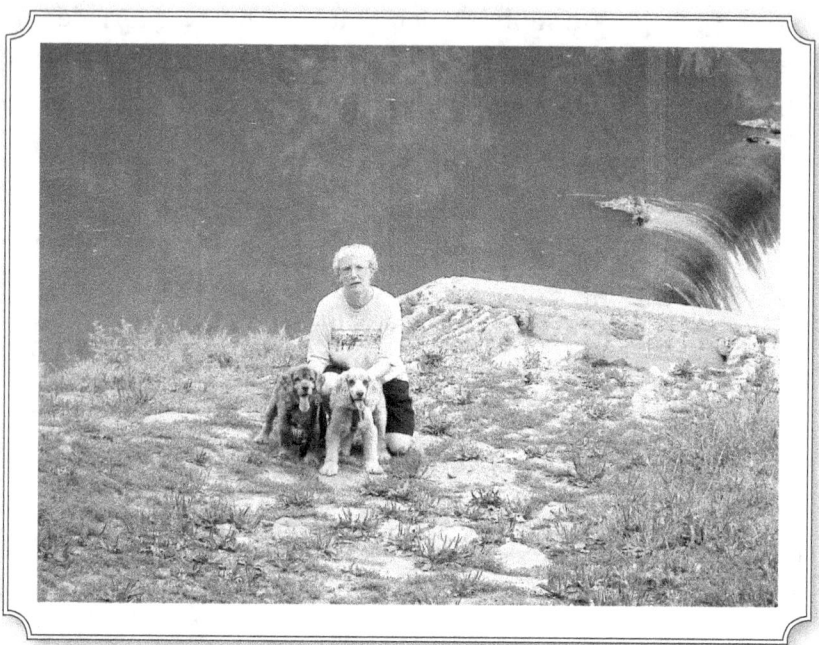

For several years, we took the cocker spaniels on a three-mile walk at Englewood MetroPark almost every Sunday morning. This is one of their favorite places to walk.

One warm Christmas morning, we walked the cockers in the MetroPark. Later that day, a family of four was walking their puppy in the park when it got loose and jumped into the river near the low dam. The man jumped in to save the puppy, and then his wife jumped in to save him. Both of the people, along with the dog, drowned as their two teenage daughters watched helplessly. This was in the same area where I had posed for a photo a few months earlier with Bubba and Barkley. I never got that close to the low dam again.

Since this was Barkley's favorite walk, we reminisced about him the first time we walked there after he crossed the Rainbow Bridge. He had last walked there about seven months earlier, and it was all he could do to finish the walk, but he was determined.

A few months after we adopted Betsy, we realized she had never done the Englewood MetroPark walk. Our adventure started out as a very peaceful, uneventful walk. We saw a deer near the walking trail, but Blondie made noise and scared it away.

On the way back, we were looking for the deer again when we noticed smoke in the woods, so we stopped to see where it was coming from. We noticed a camp fire, and then a man came out from behind a tree. He yelled at us to stop staring at him. Since we were not sure what he was doing in the woods and did not want our favorite park to be destroyed, we called the park ranger to check it out before the fire got out of control.

South Bass Island Stroll

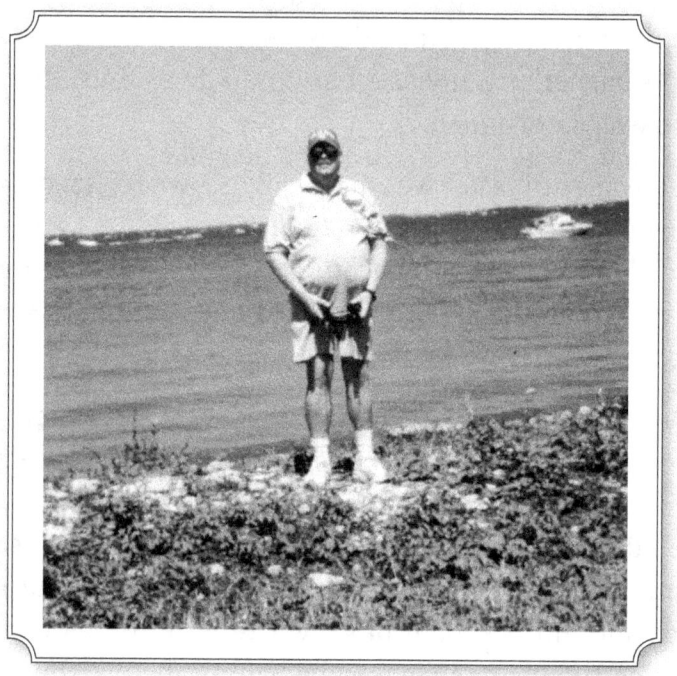

On a warm June day, we traveled to South Bass Island, near Put-in-Bay, Ohio. The small island is in Lake Erie, three miles from the mainland. A ferry provides transportation to and from the island every half hour.

A major attraction was Perry's Victory Memorial, a 352-foot-tall monument, built in honor of Admiral Oliver Hazard Perry's victory over a British fleet during the War of 1812. We paid a small fee to take an elevator ride to the top of the monument. From the observation tower, 317 feet above Lake Erie, we saw the battle site, 10 miles to the northwest.

On the ferry ride to the island, we met a group of bicyclists from West Virginia, all members of a biking club. As we waited for the ferry later that day for our return trip to the mainland, we noticed one of the cyclists arriving at the dock in an ambulance. We learned that he had fallen when his bike slipped on the rain-slicked road, after a brief afternoon shower. Hundreds of dead mayflies on the road, which we had noticed while we were walking, added to the slickness of the pavement. The cyclist had shoulder and arm injuries, and he was transported to a hospital on the mainland.

Presidential Promenade

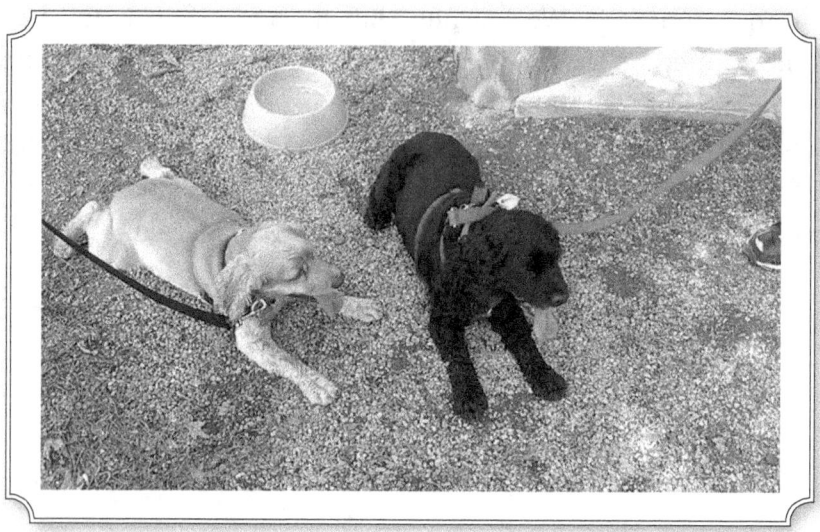

On another walking trip, we visited the Rutherford B. Hayes Presidential Center in Fremont, Ohio. We walked through historic areas of downtown Fremont, and the trail took us through the lovely grounds of Spiegel Grove, home of the Hayes family.

After the walk, we opted to take a tour of the Hayes Center and the family home. The Hayes Home is a 32-room mansion with many of the original family furnishings. Many lovely portraits of the family were on display throughout the home. We were able to see the Red Parlor, a room modeled after the Red Room in the White House, where President Hayes took the oath of office.

We toured the President's bedroom, daughter Fanny's lovely bedroom, the New Zealand Room, the Bay Room, the Oriental Room, Uncle Sardis' bedroom, the library, and several other beautiful rooms on the first and second floors of the three-story mansion.

The Hayes Museum was equally interesting, from the displays of many personal items belonging to the family to the doll house built for Fanny's first White House Christmas. Many lovely gowns belonging to the First Lady were on display, along with the official White House carriage built especially for the Hayes family.

Our tour guide explained how President Hayes walked six miles a day around the grounds of Spiegel Grove. In inclement weather, he walked up and down the massive front porch of the house, noting that 33 trips across the porch equaled one mile. We also visited the President's tomb, located in Spiegel Grove.

Wandering Around Lebanon

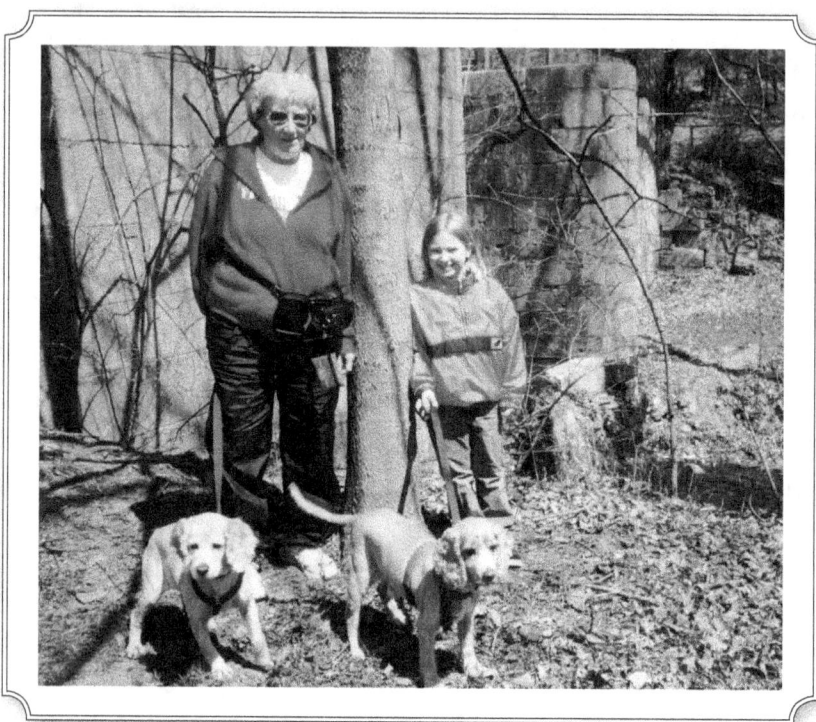

We walked in Lebanon, Ohio, several times and saw many historical and interesting sights. We especially enjoyed walking through the cemetery, where I discovered "Corwin Addition," an entire section named after my ancestors. I found several markers for ancestors I had researched over the years, including Thomas Corwin, former governor of Ohio.

On one of our walks in Lebanon, we were accompanied by Barkley and Brittany. After stopping at Dairy Queen to treat ourselves and the canines to ice cream, Brittany somehow tripped me, causing me to sprain an ankle. We were forced to eliminate the cemetery part of the walk because of a big hill.

After another of our walks in Lebanon, we visited Randy's 95-year-old Great Aunt Pearl at Otterbein Home. She was very interested in our walking stories and gave us some great advice: "Walk now, while you are still able." She had recently broken a hip and used a walker. Aunt Pearl's great advice made me realize how lucky we were to be able to walk and visit so many interesting places. I adopted a new motto: "So many walks, so little time."

Tall Ships in Toledo

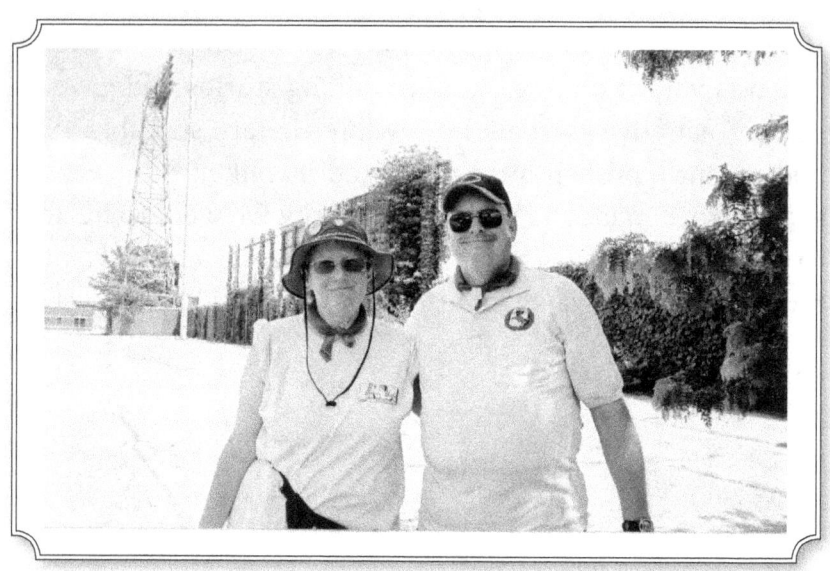

One summer, the majestic Tall Ships were docked for a week in Toledo. We decided to go see the ships and get some exercise at the same time. We meandered the length of the downtown riverfront, passing by many Toledo landmarks, including the Valentine Theatre, the Oliver House, the Erie Street Market, Fifth Third Field (home of the Toledo Mud Hens), and the Lucas County Courthouse.

The walk also included the Anthony Wayne Bridge, a suspension bridge built in 1931 and named after General "Mad" Anthony Wayne. The 1252-foot-long bridge spans the Maumee River. My friend Judith was walking with me that day. When I mentioned that I wanted to walk to the highest elevation of the bridge, she wished me luck, since she was afraid of heights.

Judith, a college secretary, was a very interesting lady I met on the trail. We walked together often, and Judith told me I could bring along as many of my cocker spaniels as I wanted to, as long as I didn't bring any children with me. Judith did not like little kids, since she was accustomed to spending her days with college students. She later surprised everyone by marrying an older gentleman she had seen walking around the campus every day. Judith explained that she knew Jerry was a "good guy" because he was a walker, so she introduced herself to him one day.

Six-County Weekend Tour

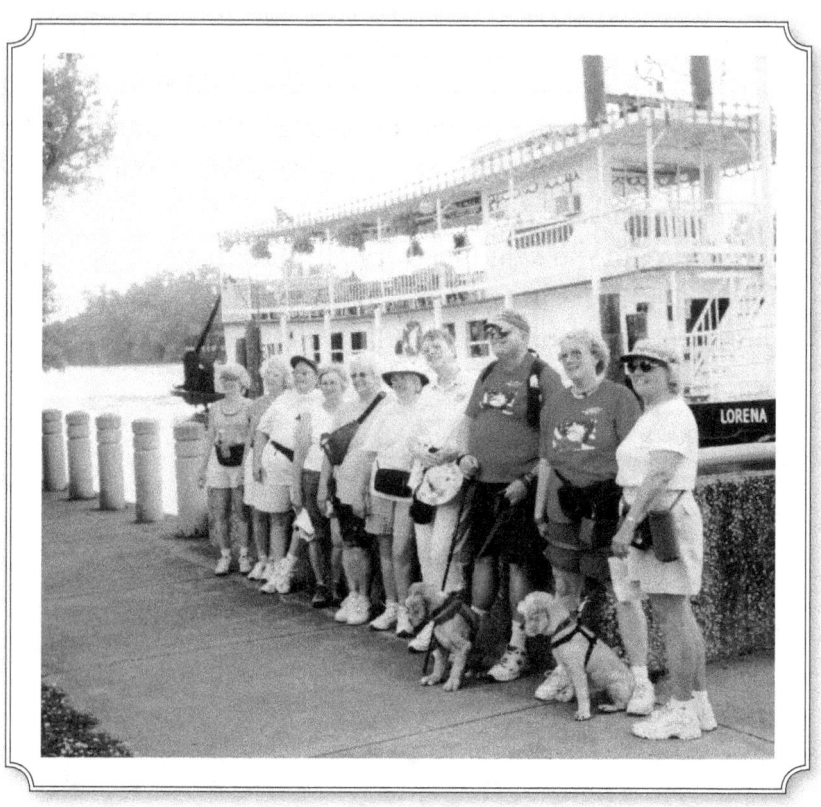

In honor of Ohio's Bicentennial in 2003, many people tried to walk in each of Ohio's 88 counties. In pursuit of our own goal, we took a weekend trip to southeast Ohio to walk in six different counties. Our first walk was in Orville (Wayne County), the home of Smucker's Jelly. The trail took us past the Smucker's factory and the historic home of the Smucker family.

In the afternoon, we walked around at a nature preserve built around a lake in Wilmot (Stark County). We met up with some friends from Toledo on the trail. They warned us that the gates at the preserve were locked promptly at 5 p.m., so we needed to be done walking by then or plan on spending the night at the preserve.

The following morning, we traveled to Steubenville (Jefferson County), the home of Dean Martin. The town was decorated with 24 murals hand-painted on buildings, including one mural featuring Mr. Martin. I was lucky enough to win a door prize at this walk, a pair of New Balance walking shoes.

In the afternoon, we joined another Toledo friend on a wooded trail in Lisbon (Columbiana County). The biggest challenge of the day was crossing a small river on a rope bridge. After walking downstream for a distance looking for an alternative trail, we decided we had two options: using the rope bridge or swimming across the river. We all successfully crossed on the rope bridge.

Our final day of the long weekend took us to Carrollton (Carroll County) in the morning and Dover (Tuscarawas County) in the afternoon. We walked with a large group of people we knew from all over the state of Ohio, and we saw areas of our state we had never before visited.

Hiking the Hoosier State

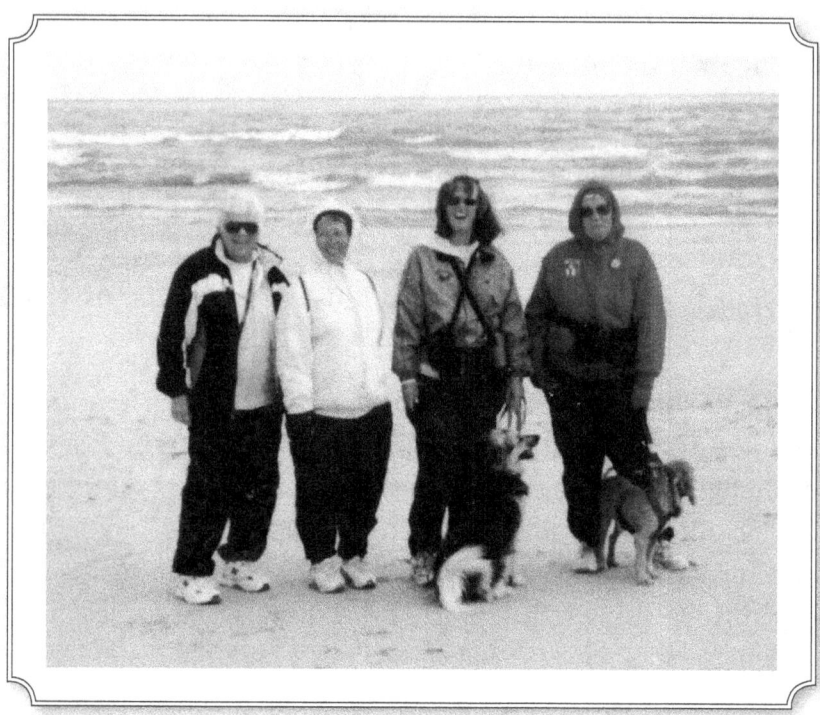

Before we moved to southern Ohio, we lived very close to the Indiana border, so we did a lot of our walking in the "Hoosier State." We were members of two Indiana walking clubs for a few years. We walked in Angola, at Pokagon State Park, home of the famous Potawatomie Inn. The trail was 12-kilometers long and quite challenging, with a lot of hills.

We walked in Fort Wayne, Indiana, many times. One of the walks started at the VA Medical Center. My Grandpa

Corwin passed away at this hospital when I was a young child, so it was full of sad memories for me. The hospital had a lot of rules. Dogs were not allowed on the hospital grounds, including the parking lot. When we took Barkley along, we parked on the far side of the lot and waited until there was no security guard in sight. We quickly got Barkley out of the car and started walking away from the hospital.

Another Fort Wayne walk went past the Botanical Gardens, the Lincoln Museum, and the historic St. Paul's Lutheran Church, with beautiful music that could be heard for blocks. One lovely spring day, we enjoyed hundreds of beautiful tulips and daffodils along the walk route.

One of our favorite walks was in South Bend. The walk was almost entirely on the campus of Notre Dame University. We tried to walk in South Bend twice every year.

We walked in Anderson, along the river walk, and past Anderson University. We also walked in Muncie, on the campus of Ball State University, our good friend Thelma's alma mater. Another summer weekend of walking took us to Tipton Lakes in Columbus, Indiana.

In the summer, we often attended the annual Pickle Festival walk at St. Joe. The 12-kilometer walk was mostly on country roads, and we visited the Sechler Pickle store along the walk route. Barkley accompanied us on this walk several times.

We also walked in Kendallville, on the grounds of the Mid-America Windmill Museum, where we saw hundreds of windmills along the trail. A walk in LaGrange, Indiana, in the heart of Amish country, also had some interesting murals and a wood carver. We also walked in Winona Lake, and after the walk we had lunch with some of our walking friends at a nice restaurant on the lake.

One weekend adventure took us to northwest Indiana. Barkley accompanied us on this very cold, rainy weekend, which included a walk along the beach at Krueger Memorial Park in Michigan City. Another walk was at the Wolf Park in Battleground. Barkley and his friend Tootsie had to wait in the car while we toured the park and looked at the wolves, since dogs were not allowed inside.

We also walked on the campus of Purdue University in Lafayette. Barkley was very cold and wet after the walk, so we took our jackets off in the car and wrapped him up in them. He had managed to get a very large burr stuck in the fur on his paw, and we could not get it out, so we ended up cutting it out when we got home.

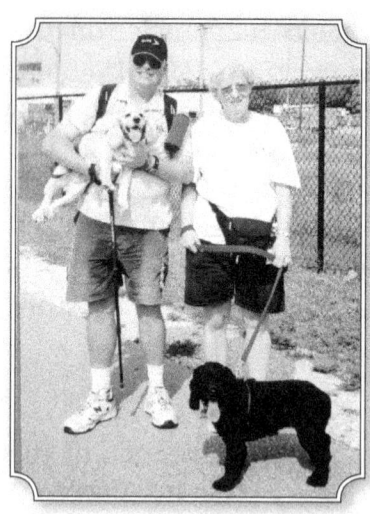

We completed a walk in Indianapolis on a very hot summer day with Blackie and Blondie. We walked under a highway overpass and noticed that someone had made a home there, complete with furniture and a box fan. Our friend Don insisted on taking a photo of us with the cocker spaniels at the end of the walk when we were quite warm and very tired.

A Kazoo in Kalamazoo

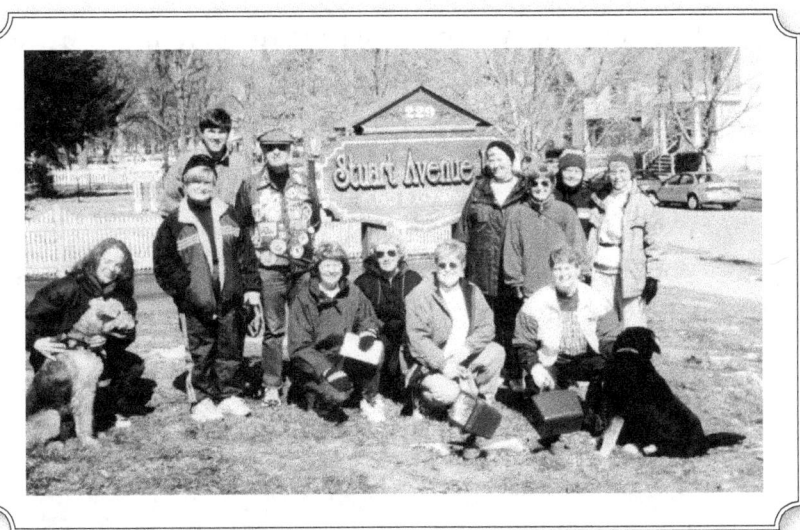

We lived very close to the Michigan border before we moved to southern Ohio, so a lot of our walking adventures took place in Michigan. A walking club there invited Randy and me to a group walk in Kalamazoo one cold March day. Thirteen walkers and two dogs (not ours) braved the cold weather to walk around the campuses of Western Michigan University and Kalamazoo Community College.

The walk started at the Stuart Avenue Inn, a historic bed and breakfast housed in two lovely Victorian homes. We were each given a plastic kazoo after the walk, along with the lyrics to the song, I've Got a Gal in Kalamazoo. We gave one of the kazoos to our young granddaughter. Her parents hated the noise so much that they told her to take the kazoo outside, and it soon came up missing.

Several times, we walked in Lansing, where our son lived for about a year. We walked past the state capital and along the river walk. We took a wrong turn on the river walk one rainy day and ended up walking a lot more than 10 kilometers. Our son was waiting for us to arrive for lunch, and we were very late.

We walked in nearby Coldwater and Marshall, Michigan, many times with Barkley and Brittany. Our friend Judith accompanied us on several of the walks.

Greenfield Village Jaunt

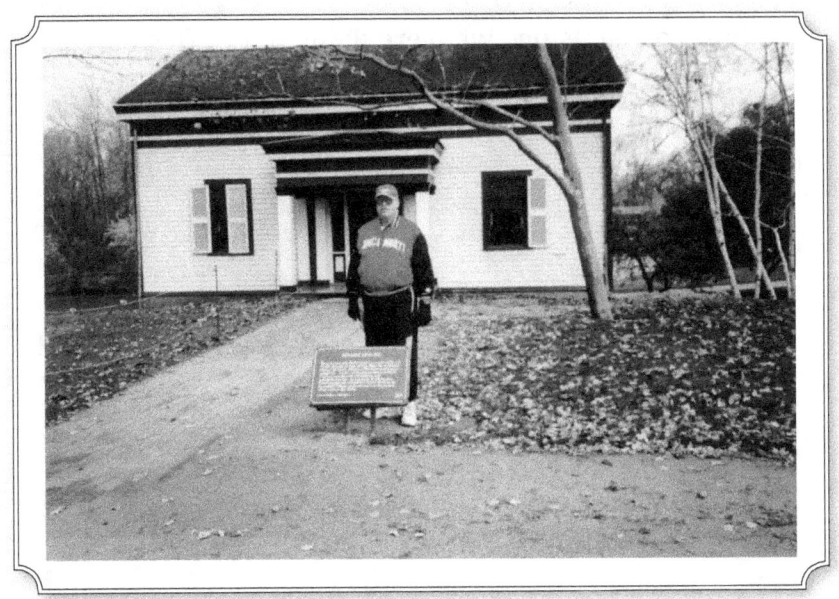

We visited Greenfield Village in Dearborn, Michigan, on one of our walking adventures. We walked around the village, touring many of the historic homes and villages located along the trail. We visited Henry Ford's birthplace, Wright Cycle Shop, Thomas Edison's Menlo Park laboratory, a covered bridge, a windmill, a glass shop, a sawmill, and a train station.

There were dozens of historic homes in the village, including the very interesting home of Noah Webster, writer of the first truly American dictionary. The village offered many forms of transportation for a small fee, including train, steamboat, horse drawn carriage, and vintage buses.

The village also featured several restaurants, gift shops, the Henry Ford Museum, and IMAX theater, which we didn't have time to visit, since we were flying out of Detroit Metro later that day, to go on another walking adventure.

Striding Around Virginia Beach

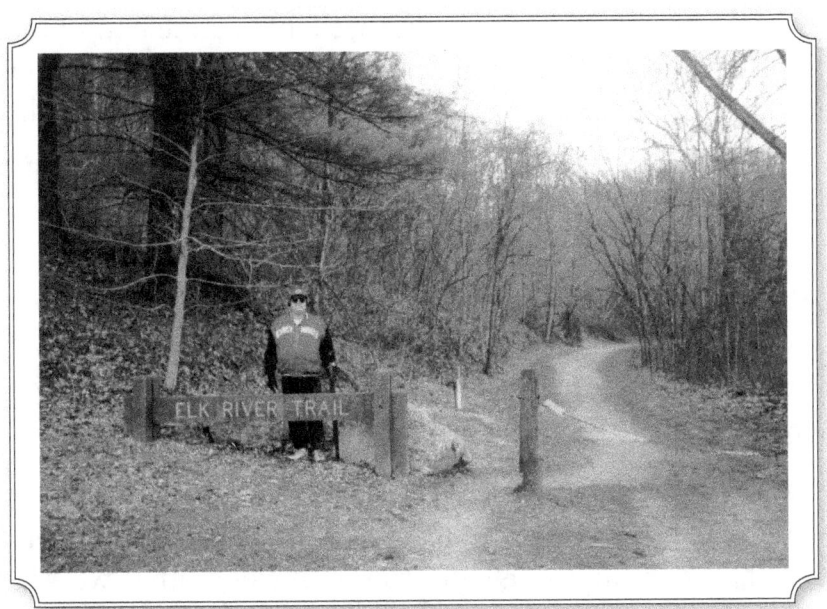

In the late '90s, our son was in the Navy and stationed at Virginia Beach. When we visited him, most of our sightseeing was done on foot. Our first visit became a seven-day, six-state walking trip.

We started our vacation in Kentucky, where we completed the two-state river walk that went from Covington to Cincinnati. We walked across three bridges on that trail.

Next, we stopped at Charleston, West Virginia, to walk at Coonskin Park. The hilly trail challenged us, but the scenery was beautiful. At the top of the biggest hill on the trail, I stopped to catch my breath and asked Randy if he had brought his cell phone. He wanted to know if I was okay, and I replied that I just wanted to be prepared, in case there were any more hills like that one!

We encountered a loose Rottweiler near the end of the last trail, the Elk River Trail. The big dog didn't really bother us, but he did follow us for a while. We were very nervous after our recent Rottweiler encounters in Bryan, and we completed the trail in record time.

Next, we traveled to Elizabeth City, North Carolina and walked along the city streets. The people there were some of the friendliest folks we met on the entire trip. The walk was mainly on the dock along the harbor, with lots of wind and seagulls.

We spent several days in Virginia with our son and his wife. The weather was rainy, but being dedicated walkers and not wanting to deviate from the agenda that we had planned months earlier, we walked in the rain. We walked along the deserted Virginia Beach boardwalk and never had to slow our pace to dodge other pedestrians. The walk started at the Atlantic Wildfowl Heritage Museum. The next day, we walked around the Rudee Inlet in Virginia Beach. The weather improved for our last walk in Virginia, in downtown Norfolk.

On the trip home, we stopped in Frederick, Maryland, to complete the most enjoyable walk of our trip with perfect weather, finally. Frederick was a very nice town with a lot of history. The entire town was filled with some flowering bushes, and the smell reminded us of cat urine, which was not at all pleasant.

We walked past the Schifferstadt Museum, through Baker and Carroll Creek Linear Park, and past Hood College. We visited Mount Olivet Cemetery, the final resting place of Francis Scott Key and several Confederate soldiers. We walked past the Hessian Barracks, under the Community Bridge, and along Frederick's "antique walk," where there were many interesting shops.

What Happens In Vegas

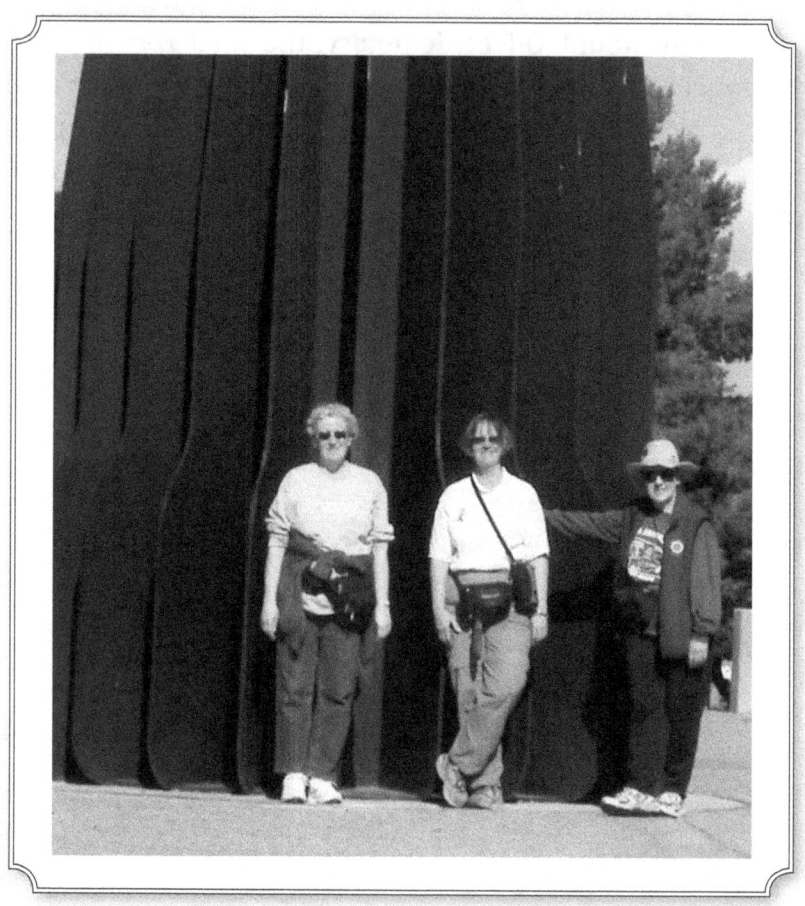

We walked around Las Vegas on five different vacations, since there is too much to see in just one or two trips. Most of the walking trails start at a small hotel, off the main drag. One trail covers the South Strip and goes past several of the casinos, including Luxor, Excalibur, New York New

York, MGM Grand, Bellagio, Caesar's Palace, Mirage, and Treasure Island.

The North Strip walk is a tour of the other end of the strip, including the now-closed Sahara, Circus Circus, Riviera, Flamingo, Stratosphere, and Stardust. We did our walking early in the morning to avoid the crowds of people on the sidewalks later in the day.

On our first trip to Vegas, we participated in a one day walk in Boulder City, Nevada. The walk was in a remote area near Lake Mead, and we were two of only 13 participants. We walked up a big mountain and through five abandoned railroad tunnels along the old Lewis Construction railroad bed. The trail was used to carry supplies during the construction of the Hoover Dam.

We shared the trail with mountain goats grazing nearby. It was very hot in the desert, and we soon ran out of water. We never saw another person or any water until we finished the walk many hours later. It was a very challenging walk and much more isolated than what we were used to.

Another walking adventure took place on the campus of UNLV (University of Nevada, Las Vegas), where we walked past the Thomas and Mack Center and the famous "Flashlight Sculpture."

We ventured outside of Las Vegas to do some more walking, after obtaining a CAT bus schedule. The buses provided relatively inexpensive transportation, once we figured out the schedule. A tourist needs plenty of time and patience to wait for the buses to arrive. We walked in nearby Henderson several times. The first trail was the Green Valley

Ranch walk, featuring beautiful homes, schools, and Paseo Verde Park in Green Valley. The landscaping and the Spanish style architecture were very interesting.

The McDonald Sun City walk, also in Henderson, is in the same area as Green Valley. We walked past more charming Spanish architecture near the beautiful Desert Willow Golf Course. The mountains were spectacular, and very close to the walking trail. The Green Valley Ranch Casino is in Henderson, and we stopped there for lunch and a little gambling.

Our sixth walk was the lakes walk, which started at a hotel on Sahara Avenue and took us past some very expensive homes, most of which were concealed by six-foot-high walls that surrounded the properties. The four small lakes along the trail are beautiful.

Orlando Adventures

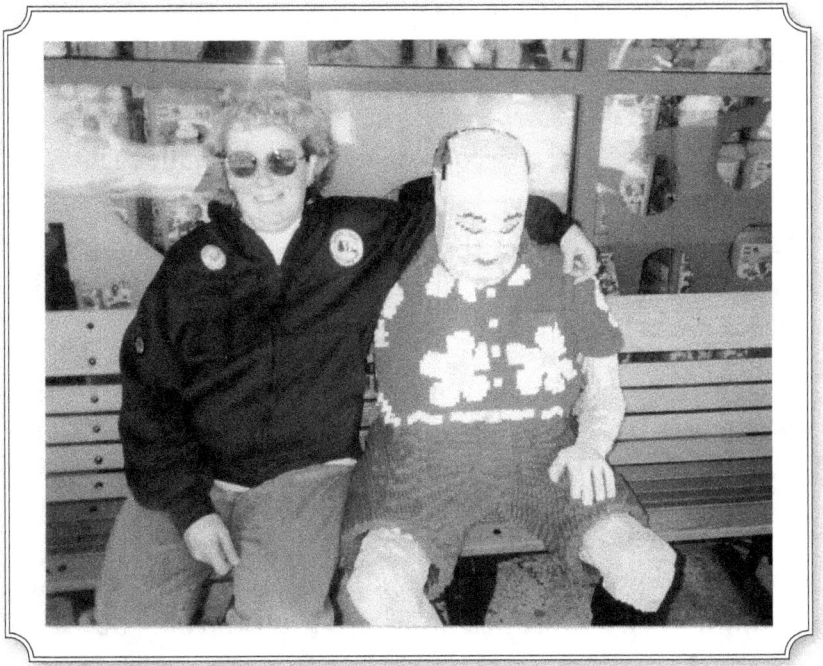

We decided to spend Christmas in Orlando one year, since our Navy son was deployed to the Middle East for six months, and the holidays at home just wouldn't be the same without him. As soon as our plane landed in Orlando, we started our walking adventures.

Our first walk was in Celebration, a fairly new city just south of Orlando, developed by Disney in 1996. The walk through the planned community was lovely, with a lot of things to see and do. While walking on the sidewalk along a busy highway, we passed an abandoned car with Ohio license plates that was stalled in the middle of the highway. A police officer pulled up next to us to ask if the stalled car belonged to us. He obviously did not believe our story about just being out for a walk, since Randy was wearing his Cincinnati Reds jacket, and the car was from Ohio. The officer followed us for a short distance.

Lake Buena Vista was one of our favorite walks. The walk started at Pirate's Cove Adventure Golf Course. We walked past many lovely hotels in the Disney area and then into the Disney Market Place. We especially enjoyed Lego Land with the life-sized Lego creations on display.

Our next walk was in Winter Park, just north of Orlando. We walked through old, stately neighborhoods, around a lake, and through the Rollins College campus.

We also walked in Maitland, and the trail took us around two lakes, past the Maitland Art Center and the Audubon Birds of Prey Center. In Winter Garden, our walk was mostly on the West Orange Trail, around Lake Apopka in Orange County.

Our final walk was in downtown Orlando. It was a very quiet Sunday morning, and most of the streets were deserted. We walked past the Orange County Courthouse and around three lakes: Lake Eola, Lake Cherokee, and Lake Davis. We saw a lot of homeless people sleeping on park benches. We noticed about 50 people gathered at an outdoor amphitheater and thought it was a church service. We soon realized they were all homeless people, and many of them were asleep. Church Street Station was the highlight of this walk, although it was a scary area. We witnessed a scuffle between two panhandlers who were arguing about the ownership of a certain street corner.

Since it was unseasonably cold, Randy was wearing his Cincinnati Reds jacket again. A homeless man stopped us and said he was a fan of Ken Griffey, Jr., one of the Reds' best players at the time. After discussing baseball for a few minutes, the man asked us for money.

Ambling Around Branson

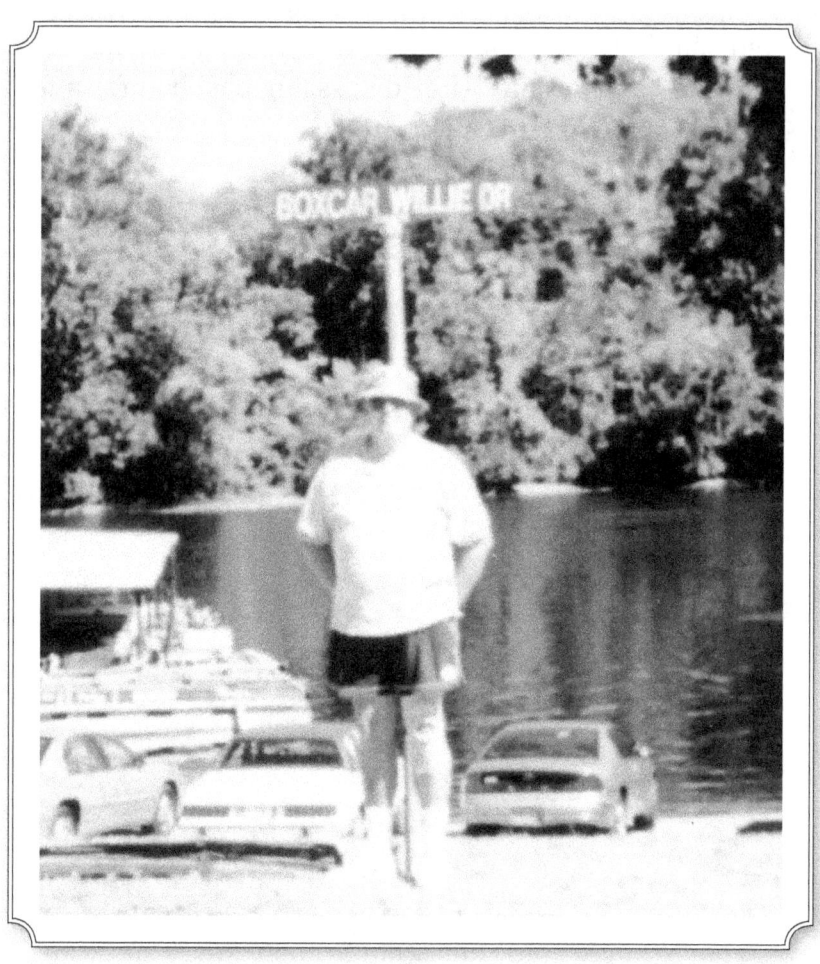

We traveled to Branson, Missouri, for a Labor Day weekend of walking events one year. On the long drive, our car was splashed by a cement truck that passed us on the highway. Cement covered the entire car, including the windshield. We had to find a car wash and clean off the cement, which had already dried. We spent more than an hour at the car wash, and when we finally arrived at our hotel, we had five minutes left to register for the evening walk.

Randy's parents lived in nearby Arkansas, and they planned to meet us for dinner after the walk. We greeted them in the hotel lobby and explained that we would be back after our walk. More than two hours later, we completed the walk and joined them for a very late dinner.

In Branson, we walked along Boxcar Willie Drive and visited several souvenir shops (tourist traps). We also walked around North Beach Park in Hollister. One of the walks was a two-state walk. It started at Dogwood Canyon in Lampe, and along the trail, we crossed the state line and walked briefly in Blue Eye, Arkansas, so we could say we had walked in that state.

The last walk of the weekend was in the Busiek State Forest in Chestnutridge, a wildlife refuge about 20 miles from Branson. The trail consisted of large rocks, which seemed like boulders to our already aching feet. It was a beautiful, scenic trail, but it proved very difficult to walk on those rocks, so we completed the five-kilometer walk and started the drive back to Ohio. We stopped for lunch at Lambert's, "Home of the Throwed Rolls," in Sikeston, Missouri.

Exploring the Crescent City

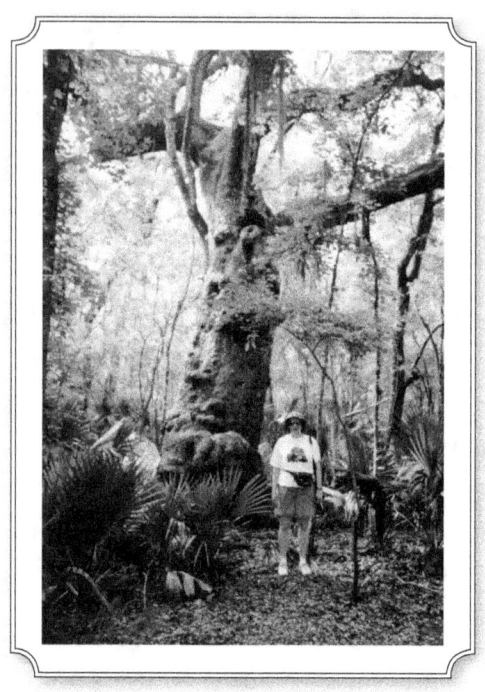

We traveled to New Orleans with my mom to visit my sister, Debbie, and her husband, Gary. As usual, we did most of our sightseeing on foot. A walking club in the area was having their annual spring walk that weekend, at the Jean Lafitte National Historic Park and Preserve. It was a lovely spring day, and we thoroughly enjoyed the five trails: Ring Levee, Wood Duck, Palmetto, Coquille, and Marsh Overlook. The first two trails were on natural surfaces, where the beautiful wild iris was in bloom, and the last three trails were on wooden walkways.

Much of the park is a swamp area, and along the trails we encountered lizards, turtles, a mother alligator and her babies, and a large snake. The snake was on the wooden walkway, and I was so intent on looking at the scenery, I almost stepped on it.

Our next walk was in downtown New Orleans, starting at Fritzel's Bar on Bourbon Street. The walk through the French Quarter was very scenic, featuring lovely old architecture. Various activities taking place along the route were an added bonus, including a belly dancer, several bands, and living statues. We shopped at the French Quarter market and walked around the Louisiana Superdome and along the river walk. After the walk, we met up with the rest of the family to take a horse and carriage ride around the French Quarter, covering some of the same area we had just walked around.

We also walked in Mississippi on this trip. Our first stop was in Gulfport, where we walked along the Gulf of Mexico, through downtown Gulfport, and around some lovely residential areas. We stopped at a drug store with a soda counter from the '50s and enjoyed some ice cream.

In the afternoon, we traveled to nearby Bay Saint Louis and walked around St. Augustine Seminary. We walked around some residential areas of the town, through two cemeteries, and around the campus of Stanislaus College. We again walked along the Gulf of Mexico on some beautiful beaches.

A few years later, this entire area was devastated by Hurricane Katrina, so we were lucky to be able to visit before the destruction.

Niagara Falls Excursion

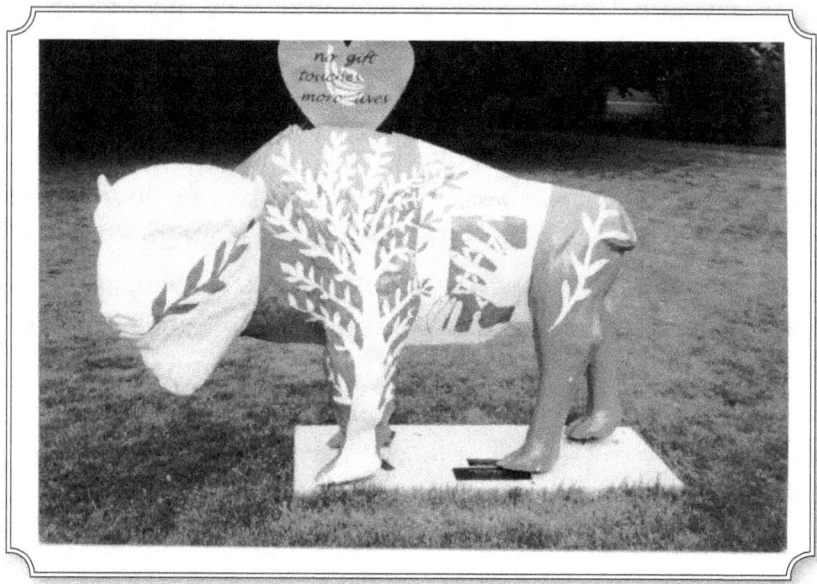

We traveled to Buffalo, New York, to visit my cousin, Cyndy, her husband John, and their two dogs, Isabelle and Maxine. On our road trip, we stopped in Sharon, Pennsylvania to walk and sightsee. Daffin's Candy Store, which featured a 700-pound chocolate turtle, was the highlight of the walk. We walked around the campus of Penn State University and past the Buhl Mansion Park and the golf course. The walk ended at Quaker Steak and Lube, where we enjoyed a great dining experience in a very unique atmosphere.

We again did most of our sightseeing on foot. Our walking adventure started on the Canadian side of Niagara Falls. We took a walking tour, "Journey Beneath the Falls," which provided a very close-up view of the falls. We walked around Dufferin Island, Goat Island, and Three Sisters Island and crossed the Rainbow Bridge to get a better view of the American side of the Falls.

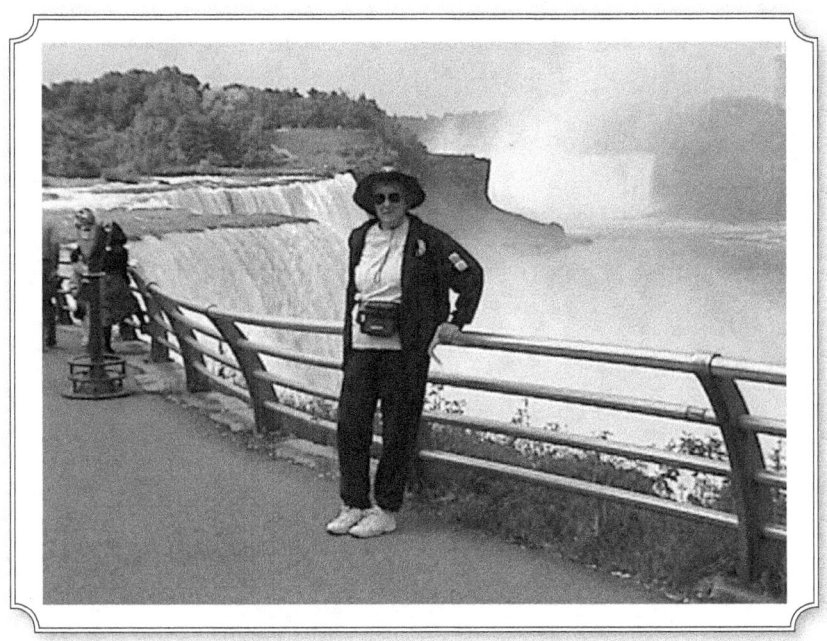

Our next day of walking started at Schoellkopf Geological Museum on the New York side of the Falls. We walked around Goat Island again and through Oakwood Cemetery, the final resting place of Annie Edson Taylor, the first woman to go over Niagara Falls in a barrel and survive. We visited the IMAX theater after the walk, saw a movie about the Niagara daredevils, and looked at a traveling display that included a replica of Ms. Taylor's famous barrel. We also walked around the Great Lakes Gardens, passed by three of the falls, and walked through historic Stone Chimney cemetery.

We walked around downtown Buffalo, including the McKinley Monument, the Erie Basin Marina, Delaware Park, and the Marine Museum. We were supposed to follow the blue buffalos painted on the sidewalks, but we sometimes strayed from the trail when the buffalos disappeared. Cyndy later told us that many of the sidewalks had been replaced recently. The walking club had forgotten to update the walk directions after the construction.

Our final Canadian walk was in St. Catharines, Ontario, a lovely, quiet town. The sixth largest city in Ontario, St. Catharines is famous for its parks, gardens, and trails. We ate our breakfast at a pancake house along the trail.

Trekking in Texas

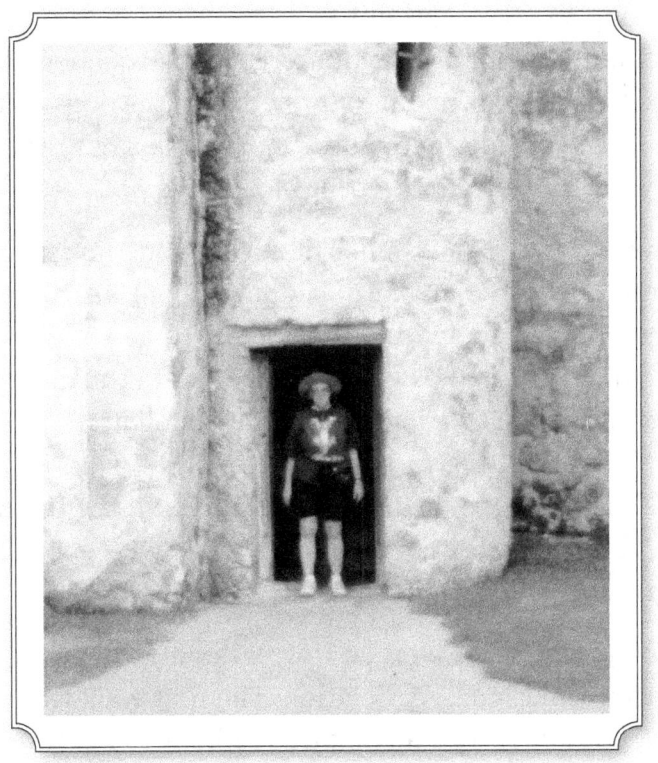

We traveled to San Antonio two weeks after 9/11, which was an interesting time to be at an airport. Our first walk was along the San Antonio river walk, and we also walked around Hemisphere Park. We passed by the San Fernando de Bexar Cathedral, a historic church built in 1748. We walked by the Bexar County Courthouse and past the San Antonio Convention Center. A highlight of the walk was visiting the Alamo.

The following day, we completed the first of three San Antonio Mission Trail walks. We walked from Mission San Jose to Mission San Juan, on the grounds of Mission San Jose National Heritage Park. The trail took us down a hike-bike trail along the San Antonio River, past the historic Espada Dam and Aqueduct. We encountered a pack of about 10 wild dogs along the trail, and we stopped until the dogs went into the woods. We saw them a few more times, but they didn't seem at all interested in getting close to us.

The other two Mission walks were on the grounds of Mission San Jose and Mission Concepcion, near the same trail where we had spotted the wild dog pack. It was a very hot October day, and as we crested a hill, I thought I saw an ice cream truck parked in the middle of nowhere. I was sure the heat was getting to me, but it really was an ice cream truck. The ice cream tasted very good, but it melted rapidly in the Texas heat. We completed the walk with chocolate ice cream stains on our shirts.

Two of the walks were in Universal City, the home of the American Volkssport Association. The first walk was mainly on a wooded country trail that was rather boring. The second walk took us through residential areas and a park and past the AVA National Headquarters on Universal City's main street. We stopped at the headquarters and had the grand tour of the very small, cramped office in a strip mall. It was interesting to see the displays and meet the office staff.

Floribama

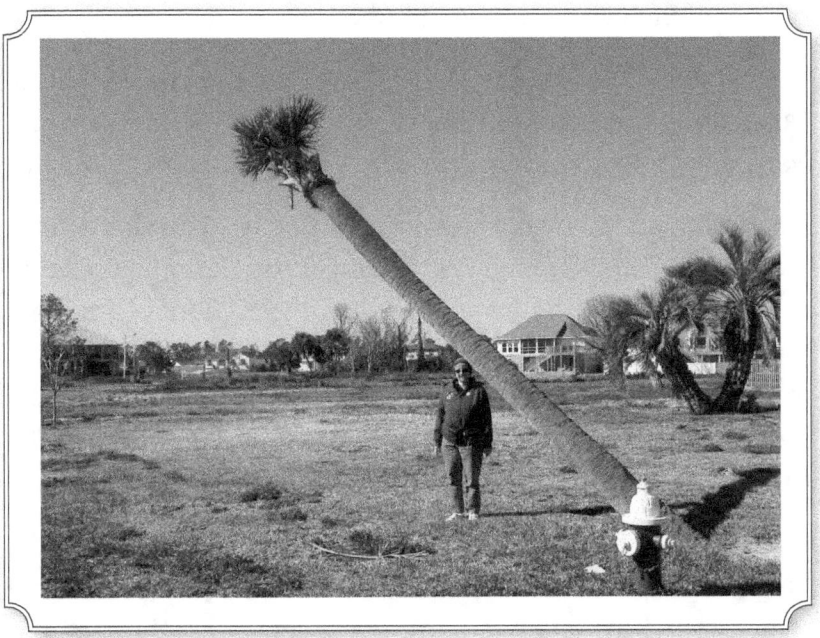

Several clubs sponsored a weekend of walking events in Florida and Alabama during Presidents' Day weekend. We attended the Floribama event four times. The first time we went to Gulf Shores, we visited Uncle Bob and Aunt Alice, who spent their winters in Alabama. They took us to Lambert's, "Home of the Throwed Rolls," in Foley. That was a very enjoyable experience, especially watching Aunt Alice try to catch a roll. Randy finally caught one for her, since my aunt's athletic abilities were almost non-existent.

Uncle Bob collected items from garage sales in Ohio during the summer and sold them at a flea market in Alabama during the winter. We went to the flea market on a Sunday morning and attended the church at the flea market that my aunt and uncle were active members of.

Many of our walks in Gulf Shores were in the Gulf State Park, along the beautiful beach. We also completed several walks in Orange Beach and at nearby Perdido Bay in Florida.

We stayed in Pensacola for an extra day to do some more walking and sightseeing. We walked at the National Museum of Naval Aviation. We saw some forts, the National Cemetery, Navy Yard, and a lighthouse. As we were walking along the walking path behind the museum, a red fox darted across the trail in front of us. Randy was very interested in the Museum, so we spent several hours inside.

We also walked around Fort Pickens, located in the National Seashore Park. We saw several Civil War fort structures. Our last walk in Pensacola was the historic downtown walk.

We left Brittany, Bubba, and Barkley at the kennel while we were in Florida. When we picked them up, we noticed that Barkley was very lethargic. At first, we thought he was just tired from all of the excitement at the kennel. He didn't want to eat, which was extremely unusual. He already had an appointment scheduled for a shot, and the vet ended up doing blood tests and changing Barkley's arthritis medication.

A few hours after the vet appointment, Barkley threw up a three-inch long splinter of wood. He fell down on the floor after vomiting and just laid there for a few minutes. I called the vet's office and was told to make Barkley eat some Vaseline in case there were more splinters inside of him. Getting a dog to eat Vaseline is no easy task, especially when the dog is sick and grumpy.

When we got the test results, Barkley's red blood count was half of what it should have been, and his white blood count was elevated. His protein level was low. The vet told us that Barkley was "in serious trouble." That was his polite way of telling us that Barkley might not survive the weekend. By Sunday, he was acting a little better and wanting to eat people food.

Barkley did recover from that episode, but his walking days were over. The arthritis had gotten really bad, and his idea of a walk was checking out the fire hydrant in our front yard and then going back to his soft dog bed.

Walking in the Desert

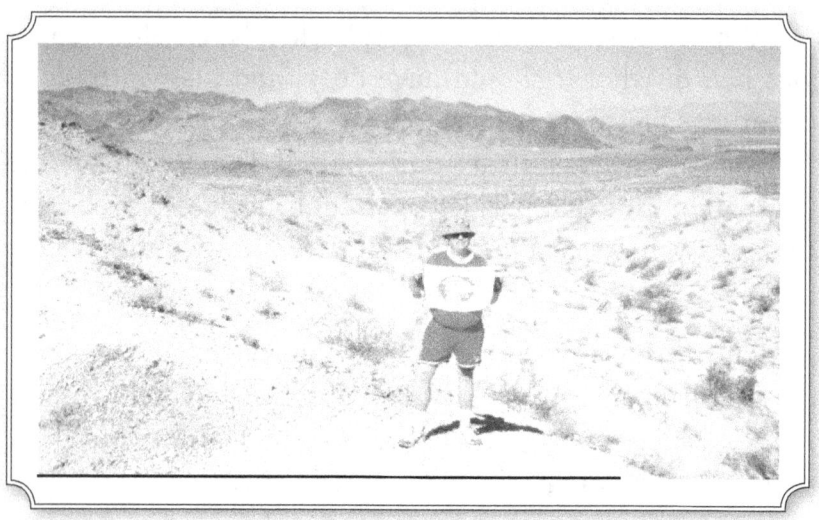

We traveled to Las Vegas several more times. We walked a lot and gambled a little. One spring, after flying to Vegas, we rented a car and drove to Laughlin, Nevada. The long drive through the desert at night was rather scary, with no stores or gas stations for most of the trip.

We stayed at the Avi Casino, owned by the Mohave Indian tribe, where all of our planned walking events started. The trails were mostly on gravel surfaces along the beautiful Colorado River. The desert is extremely warm in the spring, so we started our walks very early each morning.

Three different walking trails started at the hotel, and each trail led us to a different state: Needles, California;

Bullhead, Arizona; and Laughlin, Nevada. We saw a black and white king snake on the Needles trail and nearly stepped on it, not once, but twice!

One morning, we saw a large rolled-up rug lying across the trail just ahead of us. I was sure the discarded rug was concealing a dead body. We cautiously approached, checked it out, and found that it was just a discarded, oversized rug. Perhaps my imagination was oversized, too, or the desert heat was getting to me!

A group walk in Nevada was led by Mary, a professional tour guide with Tater Tours. The trail went through the back country around the Indian reservation, with fascinating desert scenery. Nightfall was approaching, and Mary encouraged everyone to stay with the group, since the desert is extremely dark at night. I managed to step on an inch-long thorn, and it became embedded in the rubber sole of my shoe. We stopped beside of a fire hydrant in the middle 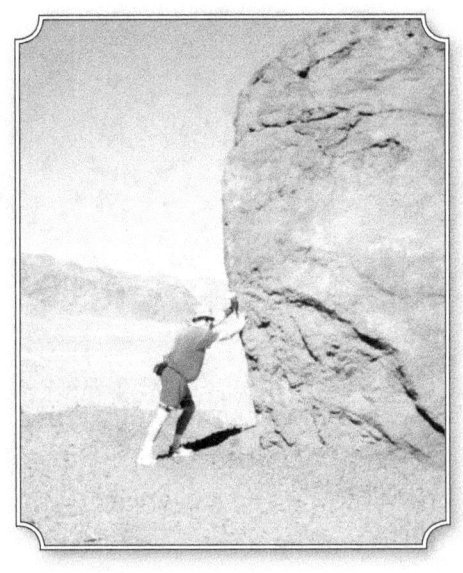 of the desert and attempted to remove the stubborn thorn. Mary retraced her steps to find us, and we finally got rid of the pesky thorn that had been jabbing my foot with every step I took. After that adventure, I always carried tweezers with me, to remove any thorns I might step on.

Star Sightings in Vegas

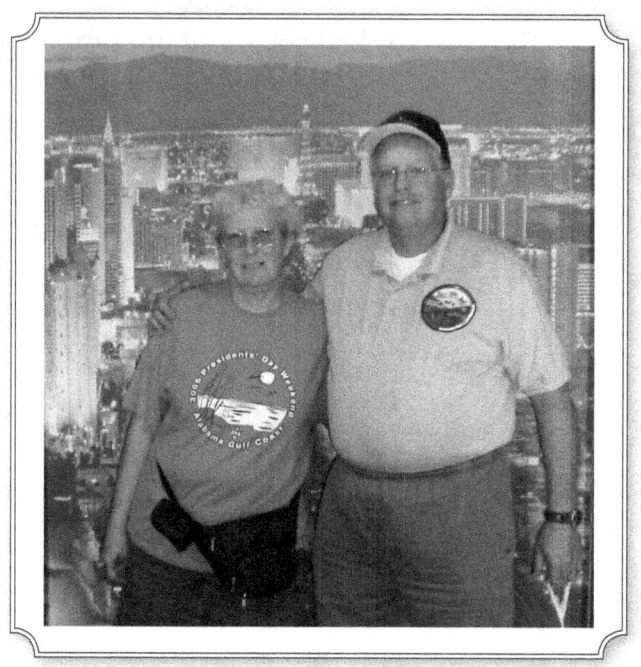

A few years later, Randy and I bought some raffle tickets to support a dog rescue we volunteered for. We won a two-night stay at the Las Vegas Hilton, and we used it to celebrate our wedding anniversary. Although we had already been to Las Vegas four times, we had never stayed at the Hilton, so I was delighted about the prize package.

It was wonderful to have two free nights at the Hilton, and all we had to pay for was airfare, four more nights at the Hilton, our meals, and boarding our four cocker spaniels at the kennel for a week.

We adopted Betsy a few weeks before our fifth trip to Las Vegas. We had not planned on adopting another dog so soon after our beloved Barkley had crossed the Rainbow Bridge. We went to the Montgomery County Animal Resource Center to check on a cocker spaniel for Columbus Cocker Rescue. That dog had been adopted, but we were told that another cocker had just arrived. We looked at the cocker and took some photos for the rescue. We soon fell in love and ended up adopting Betsy.

Two weeks later, it was time for our vacation, and we were worried about leaving Betsy. We didn't want her to think she was being abandoned again. I kept thinking about her the entire time we were walking in Vegas. Betsy was fine at the kennel, and when we got back home, she settled in like she had been part of our family forever.

Our first night in Vegas, we had gone to a square dance, and we were wearing our club shirts with the name and location of our club. After the dance, we were in the elevator at the Hilton when a very friendly and talkative man joined us. He read our shirts and noticed that we were from the Dayton area. He asked if we had ever heard of the Winters Bank in Dayton, started by his good friend, Jonathan Winters. We had not lived in Dayton very long and had never heard of that bank, although we had heard of Jonathan Winters.

The man looked vaguely familiar, and we thought he must be a celebrity if he was a friend of Jonathan Winters. After exiting the elevator, and walking around the casino area of the Hilton, we saw a poster with a picture of Chuck Woolery, the man on the elevator. He was in Las Vegas co-hosting "$250,000 Game Show Spectacular," with Bob Eubanks and

Jamie Farr. The live stage show at the Hilton had just opened two days earlier.

Randy and I obviously don't watch too many game shows on television or we would have recognized Mr. Woolery. In retrospect, we thought he seemed rather amused and pleased that we didn't seem to recognize him and ask for his autograph. He had previously appeared on "Love Connection," "Big Spin," "Scrabble," "Home and Family Show," "The Dating Game," "Greed," and "Lingo." We had not watched any of those television programs more than once or twice.

I later did some research on the Winters National Bank of Dayton, and learned that it was founded by Valentine Winters, a descendant of Jonathan Winters. The bank is now a part of JP Morgan Chase & Co. Jonathan Winters was born and raised in the Dayton area and attended college in Dayton.

We walked around the casino for a while and then decided to go up to our room. On our way to the elevator, we passed a man who looked very familiar. Randy very loudly said, "Look, it's Jamie Farr." The "M.A.S.H." star looked at us and started walking very fast in the opposite direction. Surprisingly, Mr. Farr is shorter in person than he appears on television.

Randy was a huge "M.A.S.H." fan, and we watched every episode at least 20 times. He had "M.A.S.H." shirts, "M.A.S.H." hats, and "M.A.S.H." sheets. I liked the show, but I got really tired of watching the reruns after so many years. Randy was really disappointed that he did not get to talk to "Corporal Klinger." Jamie Farr is from Toledo, yet we never saw him in person until we went to Vegas.

We were at the Hilton for several more days, but we didn't have any more star sightings.

The Windy City

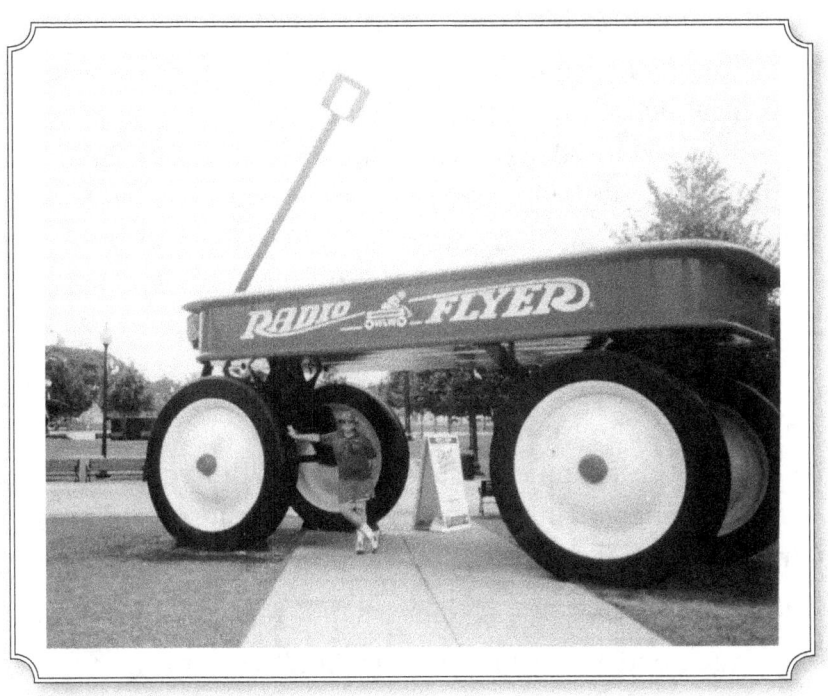

We spent a weekend in Chicago, the "Windy City." We started our walking adventures at the Chicago Cultural Center on Michigan Avenue and decided to take the Gold Coast trail along the shore of Lake Michigan, past historic homes and churches, and through Lincoln Park. We stopped to take a photo of a monument in the park and discovered that a homeless man was asleep behind the statue. This walk also took us around the campus of DePaul University and past Harry Caray's restaurant. We visited the Sears Tower (now Willis Tower), the tallest building in North America.

The next day, we walked past the marina area around Lake Michigan. The highlight of the day was the Navy Pier, a delightful shopping and dining experience. The Pier hosts interesting traveling exhibits that change several times throughout the year. We saw a Big Wheels exhibit and stopped for a photo in front of an oversized Radio Flyer wagon. The trail also took us past several of Chicago's museums, Shedd Aquarium, Water Tower Plaza, and the John Hancock Building. We walked along Michigan Avenue, which is also known as the "Magnificent Mile." We walked around the campus of Northwestern University and past Buckingham Fountain and the John Hancock building.

We walked in Oak Park and really enjoyed strolling past at least 30 Frank Lloyd Wright homes. We enjoyed the delightful old-fashioned ice cream shop on the walk route. We also walked past Unity Temple and the Ernest Hemingway birthplace and museum.

I wanted to do more walking in Chicago. Since Randy was there to attend a convention, and I didn't want to walk alone, I took a walking tour with Windy City Walking Tours. The tour started at the Sears Tower on Wacker Street and lasted about three hours, covering about four miles of downtown Chicago. The tour guide knew all of the history of Chicago and its buildings, so I learned a lot of interesting facts and walked through parts of Chicago I had not visited before.

Stepping in the South

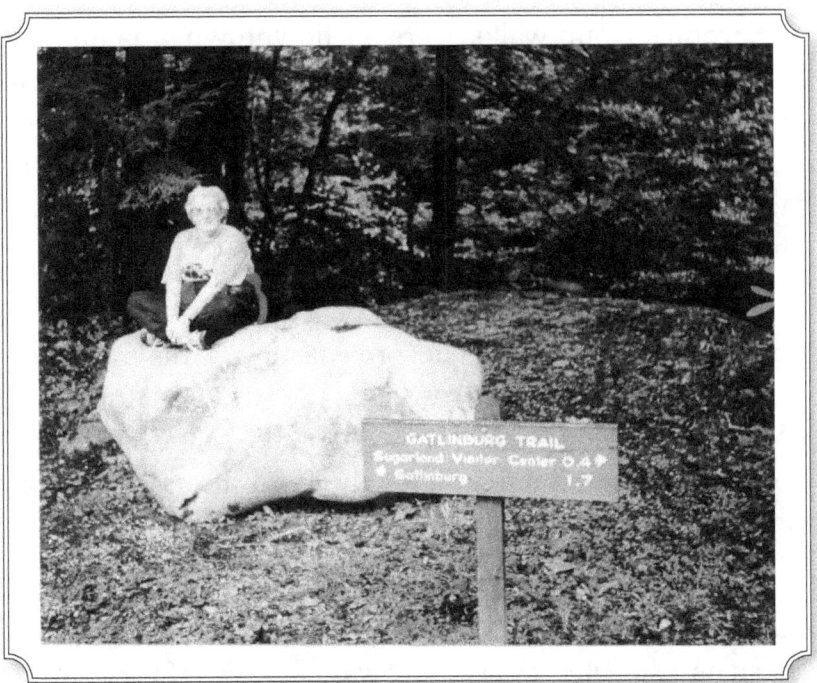

We wanted to add a few more southern states to our walking books, so we flew to Atlanta and did some walking there. We later rented a car and drove north to do some more walking and sightseeing.

We started one of our walks at the Jimmy Carter Center in Decatur, Georgia. We walked into downtown Atlanta, took a tour of Coca-Cola World, and walked past the State Capitol with its golden dome. We visited the Martin Luther King, Jr. National Historic Site, the 1996 Olympic Park, and

Underground Atlanta. We toured the CNN Studios and the Carter Library and watched a movie there after the walk. Never a fan of Jimmy Carter, Randy fell asleep and snored loudly during the movie.

Several of our walks were in downtown Atlanta, and there was a lot to see. We enjoyed the great sculptures and wonderful fountains and the Fox Theatre, famous for its premiere of Gone with the Wind. My mom and my sister had subjected me to sitting through four hours of that movie when I was very young.

Several memorable events happened on the Atlanta walks. We stopped at McDonald's for breakfast along the trail, and I used the restroom before resuming the walk. The toilet seat was not bolted down at all, and I fell off the seat, cracking my elbow very hard on the wall. Randy heard the crash through the wall, and I had a very sore elbow for a few days.

On another Atlanta walk, I was taking a photo and walked right into a speed limit sign, hitting my head. A homeless man seated on a step nearby asked if I was okay. I was fine, just very embarrassed that someone had witnessed my latest klutzy act.

We were anxious to leave downtown Atlanta after our last walk, only to discover that Randy had locked the keys in the rental car. We called the rental agency for help and then went inside a little donut shop to wait. We ate a donut, read the entire Sunday newspaper, gave a homeless man money to buy some donuts, and waited some more. Finally, a man arrived to unlock the car for us, and he didn't even charge us!

We drove to Columbia, South Carolina and walked to the State Capitol. We were given a tour of the Capitol by a very nice congressman who was working, even though the congress was on a summer break. On the outside of the Capitol building, six bronze stars mark the spots where the building was hit by artillery shells from General Sherman's cannons during the Civil War.

We saw several monuments on the building's grounds, including a monument to South Carolina's Confederate dead, a monument dedicated to the contributions and history of African Americans, and another one dedicated to South Carolina police officers killed in the line of duty. The grounds also featured statues of Senators Strom Thurmond and Benjamin Tillman. We also walked around the grounds of the Governor's Mansion and through a delightful park built around a lake.

The following day, we walked in Hendersonville and Asheville, North Carolina. The Asheville walk was on the grounds of the North Carolina Arboretum, with thousands of beautiful flowers in full bloom.

Next we stopped in Gatlinburg, Tennessee to complete the beautiful nature walk along the Gatlinburg Trail of the Great Smoky Mountains. The scenery was fantastic, and we saw a friendly couple on the trail walking their two buff cocker spaniels. We stopped to talk to them and to pet their cockers, since we were already having "cocker withdrawal."

At the visitors' center halfway through our walk, we were told that several black bears had been sighted along the trail earlier in the day. Randy wanted to walk to Cataract Falls, a waterfall on another trail, but after hearing about the bears, I said I would meet him at the car. I finished the rest of the walk in record time.

A portion of the walk was along the Sugarland's Nature Trail, and we could see the Qualla Indian Reservation from the trail. My favorite part was visiting The Happy Hiker, where the walk ended. It is the neatest walking supply store I have ever been in, and I wanted one of everything!

We drove back to Atlanta the following day, and walked around the Army base at Fort McPherson, Georgia. We enjoyed seeing all 50 state flags in front of the Forces Command building on the base and stopped for a photo in front of the Ohio flag.

Later in the afternoon, we completed a historic walk on the dirt and gravel trails at the Kennesaw Mountain National Battlefield Park. The park itself is a major Civil War battle site, and the entire walk was in the forest, with lots of hills to maneuver.

Colorado Springs Convention

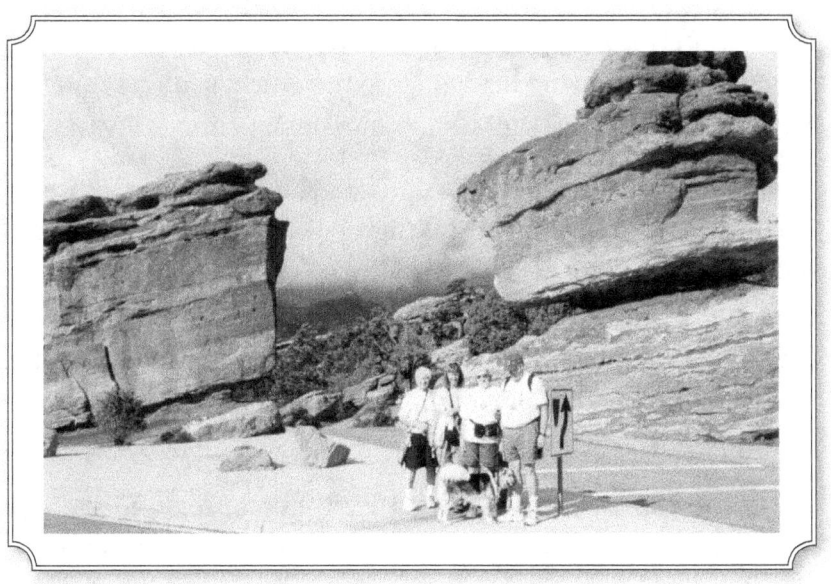

We attended the AVA 2003 Convention in Colorado Springs. Every day there was a walk in a different location, and most of the walks had over 1,000 participants. We were not accustomed to walking with so many people.

Our first walk was in Cripple Creek, formerly an old mining town and now a gambling center. We walked along a portion of the American Discovery Trail, past an old cemetery and some other historic places.

We walked at the Royal Gorge, near Canon City, approximately 45 miles southwest of Colorado Springs. We wandered through wooded areas, scenic overlooks, and rock outcroppings. We walked across the world's highest suspension bridge, over the Grand Canyon of the Arkansas River, at a breathtaking height of 1,053 feet above the river.

The Royal Gorge Bridge, which accommodates auto and pedestrian traffic, is 18 feet wide and nearly one-quarter mile long. Located near the bridge were the world's longest single-span aerial tram and the world's steepest incline railway.

We also walked at Garden of the Gods in Colorado Springs. This was a breathtaking walk with the magnificent red sandstone formations. Sculpted by wind and water erosion, the formations are estimated to be over 300 million years old. Balanced Rock, the most famous monument in the park, looks as though it might topple from its lofty perch at any moment.

At the top of the trail was a visitors' center, and we ran into one of our fellow walkers from Ohio. He was bragging about walking all the way up the mountain, yet we noticed his car in the parking lot. We were walking with Thelma, Ginny, and Tootsie, and we all just smiled at his obvious lie. The man was notorious in Ohio for cheating, often driving instead of walking.

Our next walk was in Castle Rock, a town named for its famous rock outcropping that resembles a European castle. The large rock—a cap rock that resisted erosion during the time the Colorado River was a receding ocean—stands like a sentinel above the town. The walk began at the fairgrounds and followed a river trail into the heart of the town. We walked past historical buildings, restaurants, and unique shops.

The following day, we walked through downtown Colorado Springs. We walked past the Olympic Training Center's Velodome, used for track racing and training for cyclists. Every year, more than 15,000 athletes attend training programs there, and the facilities house up to 500 athletes and coaches at one time. In downtown Colorado Springs, we walked past the Colorado Deaf and Blind School and the Colorado Springs Pioneers Museum, which was housed in the former El Paso County Courthouse. The walk continued through Acacia Park, and we ended up at the Sculpture Garden and promenade, where we saw metal figures that depicted various Olympic sports.

We also walked in Colorado City, an area rich in history, since it was the hunting grounds for several Indian tribes. We enjoyed a magnificent view of the Greenhorn Mountains and Greenhorn Peak, which rises to 12,334 feet above sea level. We also walked around tranquil Lake Beckwith.

The next walk took place at the U.S. Army's Turkey Creek Recreation Area, which is located near Fort Carson. The walk started at the OK Corral picnic shelter, one of the newer structures of the historic ranch, which was founded in 1882 for sheep and cattle ranching.

We missed the scheduled group volkswalk in Denver, so we drove there to complete a walk on our own in the "Mile High City." There was a major traffic jam on the trip there, and the entire town was a huge mess, with trash all over, due to a festival that had just ended the day before. We walked along the river, past the Capitol building, Coors Field, and Pepsi Field.

On the plane ride home, we sat next to a Boy Scout troop from Atlanta. They had been camping and hiking in Philmont, New Mexico, for 16 days. The troop leader told us that they had hiked 64 miles during that time. Randy and I had walked

66 miles in just seven days, so I felt like that was quite an accomplishment for "old" people like us!

After arriving home, I took Brittany, Bubba, and Barkley for a walk, and it seemed strange to be walking on flat, smooth, paved surfaces in Ohio after all of the challenging walks we had completed in the past week. It seemed very hot and humid in Ohio, compared to the pleasant temperatures in Colorado.

Champaign, Illinois

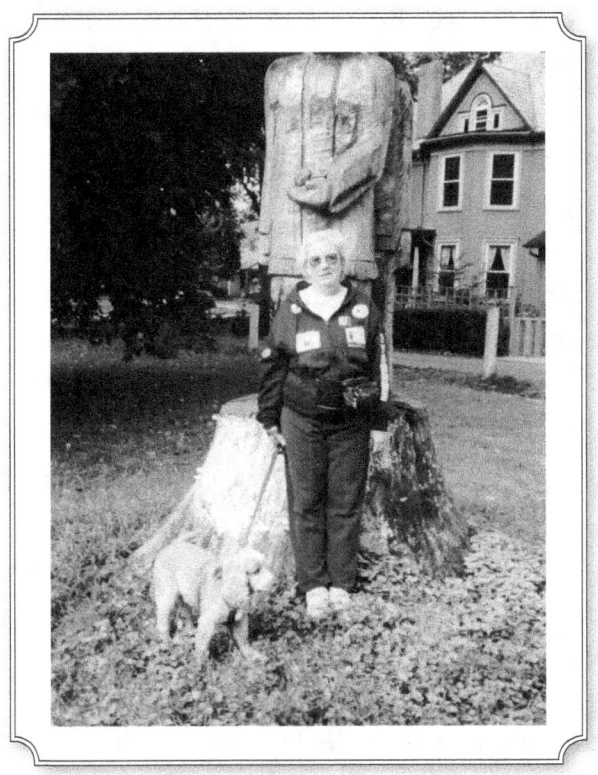

We lived in Rantoul, Illinois in 1975 when Randy was in a training squadron at Chanute Air Force Base. We decided to travel back to the area 25 years later and spend a weekend walking around and seeing the sights. We drove past the house we had lived in as a young married couple.

A walking club had organized a Marathon Walking Weekend. The first event was a guided group walk at Lake of the Woods Park in Mahomet. Mike was the best tour guide I have ever encountered, stopping to tell the group about native trees and plants. He allowed the group to stop for restroom breaks, although it took about 20 minutes for everyone to use the one outhouse we found along the trail. If someone fell behind, Mike stopped until they caught up, and he made sure everyone was having an enjoyable walking experience.

Lake of the Woods featured a waterfall, a covered bridge, and a suspension bridge, and we walked over each bridge twice. There was also an old one-room schoolhouse and a museum to tour after the walk. We enjoyed a box lunch at Pells Park after our walk, and it was fun to picnic outside on a beautiful, sunny day.

After lunch, we walked in Paxton, Illinois with two other couples. We had a great time walking, talking, and stopping for ice cream. Joy, one of our walking friends, found a little bike on a trash pile that was perfect for one of her grandchildren, so she picked it up and carried it for many miles. She couldn't pass up this great freebie. Another walker finally came along in his vehicle and gave the little bike a ride back to the starting point.

The next morning, we dodged raindrops as we walked at Homer Lake Park, near Champaign. Once again, Mike guided our tour, and since the trails were wet and slippery from the morning rain, he made sure everyone

got down the slippery slopes safely. Mike had many more interesting facts to share with us about the trees and plants. After the walk, most of the group changed out of their muddy shoes and socks in the parking lot, always prepared with a car full of spare shoes and socks.

In the afternoon, we participated in a walk around Champaign, a town we had visited several times when we lived in Illinois. Many of the walkers had lunch at Taffies restaurant, but we opted to eat in our car since Barkley was with us. As a result, we walked most of the trail by ourselves, since everyone else was still eating. Much of the trail was in the Kaufman Lake Park.

After our walk, we went out for dinner, so we left Barkley in his crate in the hotel room, quite certain he would fall asleep. When we returned, we were told there had been complaints that Barkley was barking and bothering people. The hotel manager went in the room to check on him, and decided Barkley needed the lights and television on. That did not help, since Barkley never watched television at home. After that experience, we always left Barkley in the car when we went out for dinner. He was fine in the car, since he did so much traveling with us and was used to being left in the car.

Hardy's Reindeer Ranch

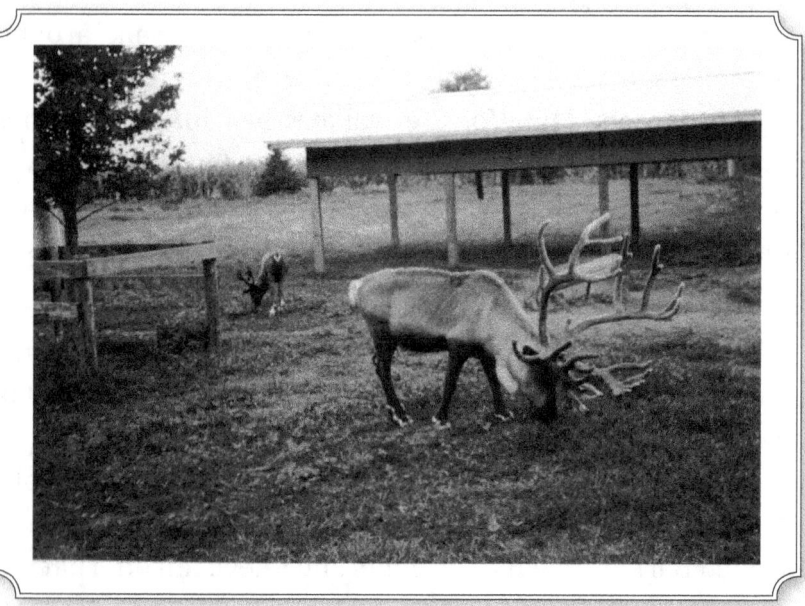

After our walking adventures, we visited Hardy's Reindeer Ranch in Rantoul, Illinois. The Ranch offers the Reindeer Experience Tour, which begins with a hayride to see the reindeer. We were able to pet the reindeer, give them a treat, and have a photo taken with the amazing animals. Klondike, Flurry, and Mistletoe were some of the most popular of the friendly reindeer.

The ranch was started by the Hardy family in 1995, with a few Christmas trees and a pair of reindeer purchased from a Michigan farmer. The two reindeer cost approximately $5,000. The Hardys later purchased more reindeer, and these animals were flown on a 747 jet from Alaska. The journey from the North to their new home in Illinois took thirteen hours. The reindeer can only be flown in the spring, before their new antlers appear. It is very difficult to transport them with antlers, as the racks get quite large.

Both male and female reindeer have antlers, and in the summer, the antlers become covered with soft velvet fuzz. The reindeer with the larger antlers tend to become the bullies of the herd, often trying to take food and treats from the others.

Until 1997, only Alaska natives were allowed to own Alaskan reindeer, so the Hardys had to obtain special permission from the Bureau of Indian Affairs. The Hardys raised their own herd after purchasing the reindeer from Alaska, and there is an average of five calves born on the farm each year.

After the tour, we visited the Country Barn Gift Shop, which was heated by an old potbelly stove. Unique Christmas ornaments, gift items, and tasty treats, including homemade fudge and cookies, were available in the gift shop. The ranch also offers the Fall Corn Maze, which encompasses 10 acres. The Maze features a different theme each year and takes from one to three hours to complete.

Another unique feature of the ranch is the Western style banquet hall with seating for 150, featuring a Western saloon with a 100-year-old wooden bar. A delicious chuck wagon dinner, including Texas barbeque brisket, calico beans, corn bread, and sweet and sour slaw was served on tin plates. Beverages were served in tin mugs, and we were given bandanas to use as napkins.

After dinner, we enjoyed the live music and comedy acts.

Historic Shaker Village

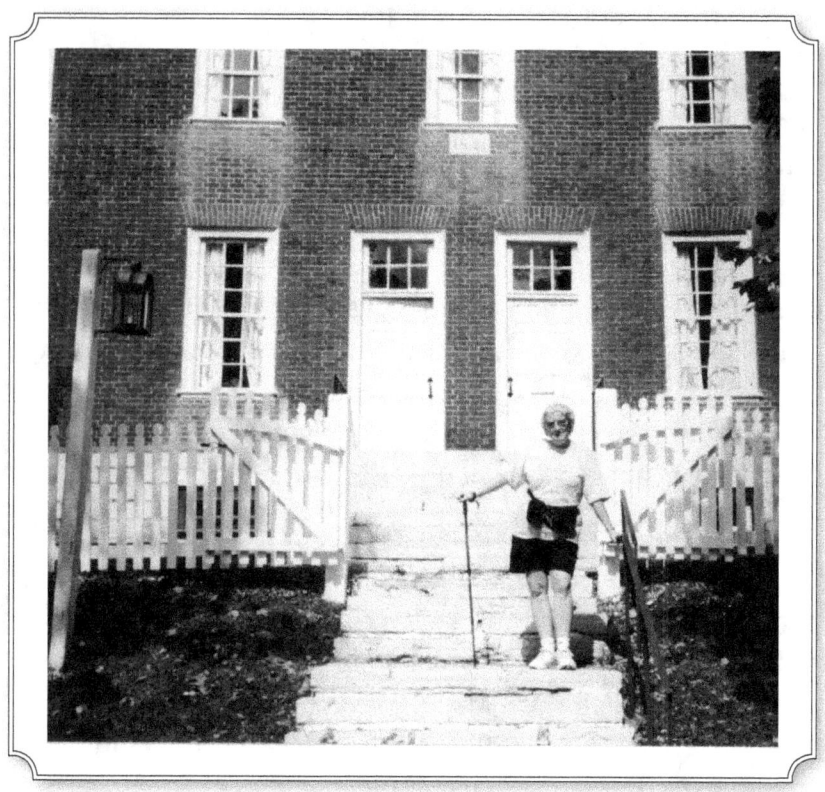

We spent an enjoyable weekend walking around Shaker Village in Pleasant Hill, Kentucky. Our first walk was delightful, in spite of the rain and the extremely challenging hills. After a wonderful buffet lunch of cold meat, cheese, and thick-sliced bread, we walked around the village and toured the buildings.

In the evening, we gathered at the village church for a wonderful music interpretation program. The program was presented by a very talented lady, who explained the Shaker traditions and sang some beautiful old Shaker hymns. After the program, we moved to the dining hall, formerly the trustee's office. A transformer had blown in the village, so we ate our dinner by candlelight, which added to the Shaker atmosphere.

The next morning we joined a guided group walk, led by the village naturalist, a very knowledgeable man who stopped often to share interesting information about the village's trails, flowers, trees, and grasses. At the halfway point of the walk, we enjoyed a delicious box lunch, and then we continued on the other half of the walk with the naturalist.

Gettysburg Bus Trip

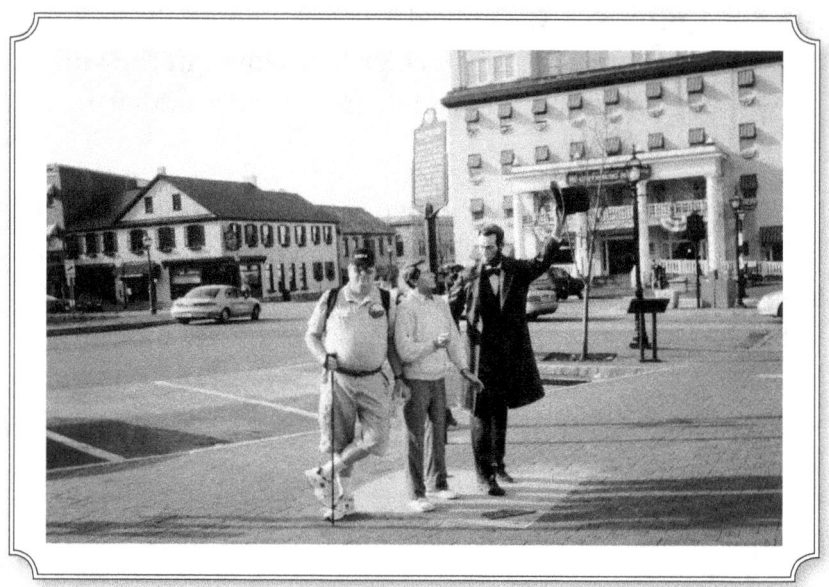

We took a bus trip to Gettysburg one spring with the Wandering Wheels Volkssport Club. We attended the Atlantic Region Conference and did two great Civil War walks in Chambersburg and one walk in Westminster, Maryland.

All of the walkers were very anxious to get off the bus and start walking, so a rule was made that, on alternate days, the back of the bus was unloaded first. A few of the walkers reminded me of the way children behaved in elementary school.

We spent several days in Gettysburg and completed all three of the historic Civil War walks. Each walk took us through the battle sites in chronological order. Day one took us to Seminary Ridge, Oak Ridge, and Barlow Knoll. Day two took us to the site of Lincoln's Gettysburg Address, the Jennie Wade house, Culp's Hill, and Spangler's Springs.

Day three's walk had a 15-kilometer option, and we were among a handful of brave walkers to complete the extra distance. The trail took us to Little Roundtop and the site of Pickett's charge. We walked through the National Cemetery. A lady in our group really needed to use the restroom at the cemetery. When several of us approached the restroom, we were greeted by an employee doing some cleaning. The man explained that the National Park opened for the season the following day, so we should come back then. He would not let us into the restroom.

There was an optional ghost walk one night. I decided to do that, instead of going to dinner at a nice restaurant with the group of walkers. The ghost walk took us through some of the Civil War sights we had seen during the day. The guide told us several ghost stories about the area. We spent about an hour inside of the Jennie Wade house looking for ghosts, although I never saw any. Jennie Wade was the only civilian casualty of the Battle of Gettysburg. It was an interesting adventure, although several of my friends thought I was crazy for giving up a nice dinner to look for ghosts in Gettysburg!

We stopped at the Boyd's Bear Country Outlet Store on the trip home. It was interesting, even though I was not a bear collector. I did buy a stuffed Boyd's dog at the store. The outlet featured three floors full of teddy bears, which were displayed by theme, and a food court on the lower level.

There was also a museum where visitors learned about the history of Boyd's Bears. The store closed in 2011.

The evening that we returned from Gettysburg, we were walking the cocker spaniels in our neighborhood when Brittany had a seizure in the middle of the street. We picked her up and moved her to the grass. There was a sign in the yard that said, "No dogs." The homeowner came outside to see why there was a dog in his yard. When I explained that the poor cocker was having a seizure, the man stomped back into his house. He obviously was not a dog person!

Soon after the Gettysburg trip, we noticed Brittany had become deaf. It may have been happening without us noticing, and being away from her for a week made the problem very obvious. We taught her American Sign Language, and she caught on very quickly.

Atlantic City Convention

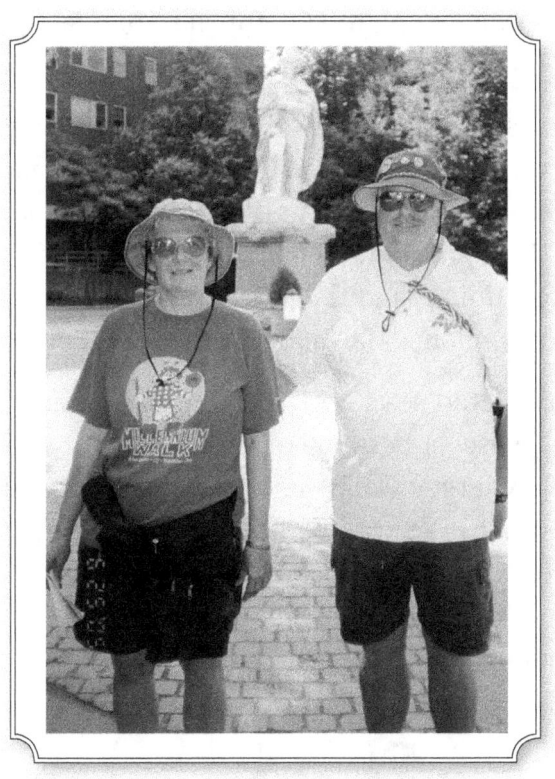

We traveled to Atlantic City, New Jersey, for the 2005 American Volkssport Association Convention. We completed a very enjoyable evening walk on the Atlantic City Boardwalk. We passed a lighthouse, Ripley's Believe It Or Not Museum, Brighton Park with the New Jersey War Memorial, Planet Hollywood at Caesar's Palace, and Kennedy Plaza. We walked along the beach for a distance. After the walk, we tried our luck at some of the casinos.

Our next walk was in Camden, along the waterfront on both sides of the Delaware River. We passed by the New Jersey State Aquarium and the Battleship New Jersey and walked around the campus of Rutgers University. One of the highlights of the walk was seeing the Campbell's Soup factory, with the oversized Campbell's Kids statues in front of the building.

We crossed the majestic Ben Franklin Bridge, with an awesome view of the Philadelphia skyline. The walk continued in Philadelphia and took us past the Betsy Ross House, Fireman's Hall Museum, Benjamin Franklin's burial site, the Constitution House, and the Jefferson Declaration House. We visited Independence Hall and saw the Liberty Bell.

We completed a walk in Trenton, New Jersey, where we had a police escort because the walk was not in a safe area. Our last New Jersey walk was in Haddonfield, a picturesque Victorian town. We walked past the discovery site of the first nearly complete dinosaur skeleton, excavated in 1858. The town is filled with Quaker history, as well as dinosaur memorabilia.

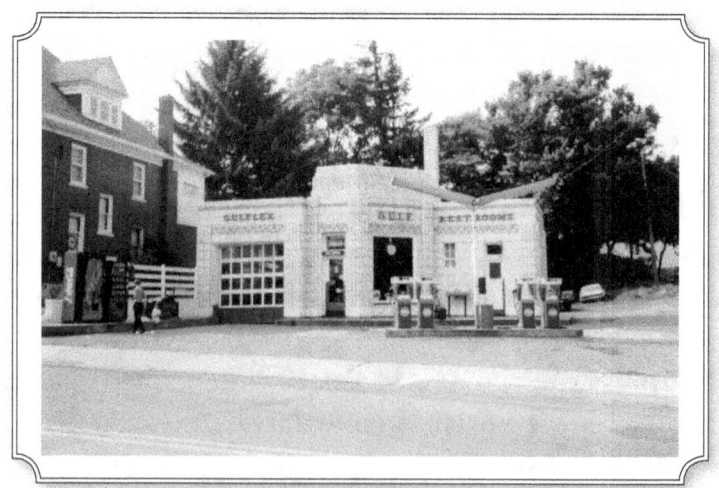

We walked in Baltimore, Maryland, on the trails through Leakin Park. We also walked in Bedford, Pennsylvania, along part of the historic Lincoln Highway. Bedford is a very quaint, old fashioned town. We walked past a Gulf Station from the '50s, and it was still open for business.

Another interesting walk was in New Hope, Pennsylvania. The trail took us past Victorian homes, antique shops, a steam train, and a mule powered barge on the Delaware Canal towpath.

Atlantic City was devastated by a hurricane a few years after we walked there. Since the same thing had happened in New Orleans and Pensacola a few years after we visited, our son suggested that perhaps we should not visit any more hurricane-prone areas of the country.

Walking in Washington, D.C.

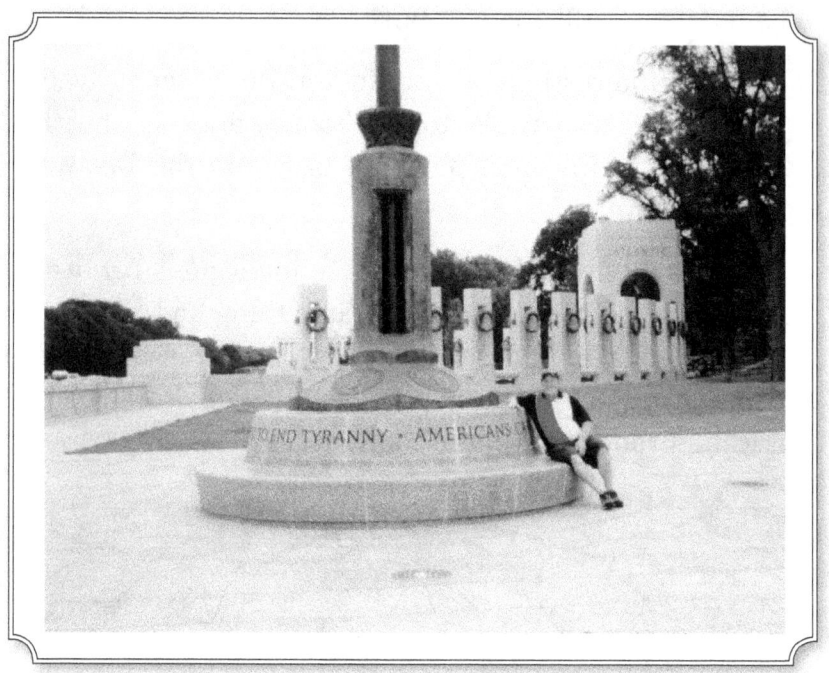

Our son Casey moved back to Virginia, so we did some walking in new locations on our next visit to his house. We stopped along the way to walk in Pittsburg, Pennsylvania. The trail took us through Schenley Park, and we walked up a very large hill.

Casey accompanied us on most of our walks. The first one was in Annapolis, passing by the Maryland State Capitol Building. We really enjoyed visiting the Naval Academy. Since Casey had served in the Navy, the Academy was especially interesting to him.

We also walked about nine miles around Washington, D.C. and visited all of the popular tourist sites with our son and his wife. Casey was wearing a brand new red, white, and blue polo shirt. A few minutes into the walk, a bird dropped his load on the shirt, splattering it all over the white part, so it was very noticeable.

Randy and I had both visited the nation's capital as young children. We were surprised to see snipers with assault rifles positioned on top of the White House. When we visited in the '60 s, the White House was open to the public for daily tours. This was during the Camelot era with the Kennedy family.

We also walked in Winchester, Virginia, the location of one of the forts built by George Washington. We passed by a grist mill, Stonewall Jackson's Headquarters Museum, the Winchester National Cemetery, and the Handley Library.

Our last walk was in Frederick, Maryland. The historic town still had the distinct cat urine odor we had remembered from our previous visit a few years earlier. We were once again reminded of why we are dog lovers, not cat fanciers!

Acknowledgements

I would like to acknowledge Columbus Cocker Rescue for providing us with some of the best walking partners ever: Blondie, Brandon, Beezus, Buffie, Brownie, and Braggs. To see all of the great cocker spaniels currently seeking furever homes, visit the website www.columbuscockerrescue.org

I would also like to recognize two wonderful Ohio animal shelters. Defiance County Humane Society provided us with our first two canine walking partners, Brittany and Barkley. We adopted Betsy, another great walking pal, from Montgomery County Animal Resource Center.

I would like to thank the family in Bryan who sold Bubba to us for a small amount of money. We didn't realize at the time that Bubba was heartworm positive. He was able to overcome the disease and serve as our walking partner for twelve years.

Many thanks to our good friend Judith, who accompanied us on a lot of our walking adventures in northwest Ohio. She never once complained about sharing the backseat of the car with the cocker spaniels.

Special thanks to our wonderful friend Thelma for sharing so many walking adventures with us. Thelma was responsible for finding Blackie for us to adopt after Brittany passed away. "Aunt" Thelma will forever be Blackie's favorite walking partner.

About the Author

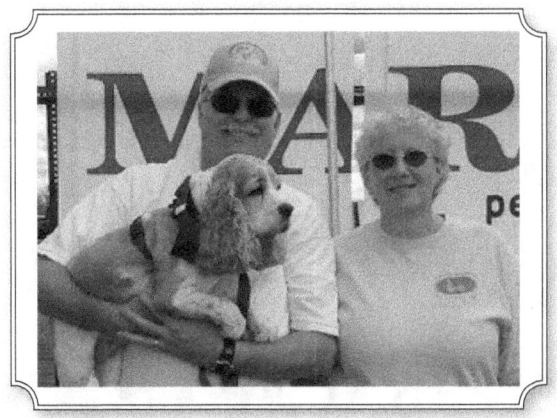

Becky Corwin-Adams was born in Defiance, Ohio. Becky is a wife, a mother of two sons, and "MawMaw" to four grandchildren. She currently shares her home with seven cocker spaniels.

As a child, Becky had one cocker spaniel, dozens of cats, chickens, and a variety of "pocket pets." She started writing stories about her pets at an early age. Becky is a freelance writer and columnist for The Farmland News and the author of *Cast-Off Cocker Spaniels*. Becky volunteers for Columbus Cocker Rescue as a foster parent, transporter, and Ebay seller.

Becky has been an avid reader since childhood. She especially enjoys reading Amish fiction, mysteries, and dog stories. When Becky isn't reading or writing, she enjoys crafting and walking with her cocker spaniels. She has had dozens of her original craft patterns published in various craft magazines.

Cast-Off Cocker Spaniels

by Becky Corwin-Adams

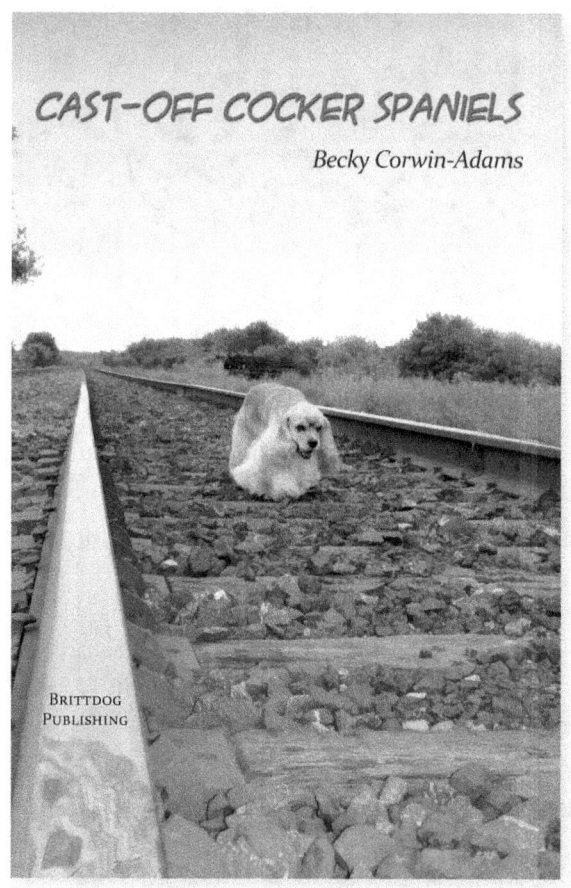

The perfect book for any Cocker Spaniel lover!

Excerpt: Nine-year-old Rags was found roaming the streets as a stray. When she landed at the shelter, she needed six baths to free her from the oil in which she was covered. Her little rear had no fur, and the skin in that area was as tough as leather. Her issues were severe, including water-filled blisters on her feet and legs.

Poor Rags was the saddest-looking cocker I had ever seen. Her eyes were downcast and droopy, and the fur around them was gone. She certainly was not very attractive.

For many long months, we treated Rags with antibiotics, and we bathed her three times a week with medicated shampoo. She was a good patient, never complaining, even though she had to soak in the bathtub for 10 minutes each time.

Finally, our efforts paid off, and a new dog emerged. At adoption events, people commented on Rags' beauty and her soulful face. This was progress! Now, our task was to convince some special person to look beyond her age.

Does Rags find a home? Buy the book to find out! Proceeds from the book are donated to cocker spaniel rescue.

Cherished Cats
and Childhood Capers

by Becky Corwin-Adams

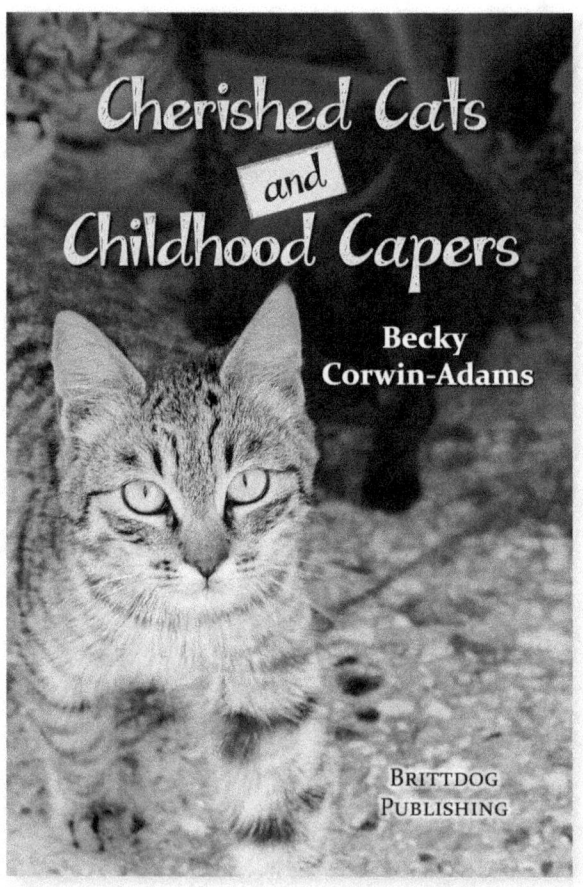

Life was never boring in Defiance!

Excerpt: "Our class went to the school library for a research project. As I was looking for a book, a note that was folded up like a football flew over the top of a six-foot-high bookshelf and landed at my feet. It was a request for my friend Cindy and me to go on a double date with Randy and his best friend, Tim.

The following day, a five-pound bag of sour balls mysteriously appeared in my locker, along with another note requesting a date. I found out where Randy's locker was and returned the candy, along with a note saying that Cindy and I had to work on Friday night, so we could not go on a date with them.

A day or two later, the persistent guys asked where we worked, and I told them we worked at Murphy's in Defiance. (I actually did work there, but Cindy didn't have a job.) I thought that was the end of them, until they showed up at Murphy's on Friday night and tried to talk to me while I was working. I didn't even know Randy's name yet. He had been signing the notes with his nickname, "Preacher Boy."

Randy found out where I lived, and on Good Friday, he dropped by my house unexpectedly. When I opened the door, with my hair full of bright pink plastic curlers that were as large as orange juice cans, there he was, asking me to join him for a cruise through downtown Defiance..."

Did Randy's persistence pay off? Read the book to find out.